BeYOnd
dieting

Naturopathic solutions
for a slimmer you and
a healthier family

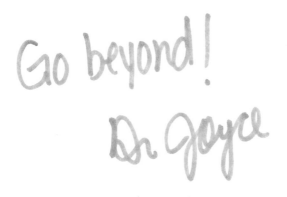

Dr. Joyce Tellier Johnson BSc., ND

CONTENTS

*"You have to stay in shape. My grandmother, she started walking
five miles a day when she was 60. She's 97 today and we
don't know where the hell she is."*
Ellen Degeneres, comedienne

INTRODUCTION

It's a fact. Obesity is now a major epidemic all across North America.

More than 30% of US adults are obese, according to results from the
1999-2000 National Health and Nutrition Examination Survey
(NHANES). The 2004 Canadian Community Health Survey proved
that Canadians are not far behind with an obesity rate of 23%.

But statistics can't show the frustration, shame and embarrassment
felt by most individuals who are overweight or obese. Whatever anyone else says or does, YOU know your body and you KNOW how you
want to be. How many pounds would you have to lose to feel like the
REAL you? Do other members of your family also want to lose weight
and keep it off?

"But it's HARD to have a healthy lifestyle." "I'm too BUSY!" "Healthy
is BORING!"

Beginning another weight loss program or making another New
Year's resolution to get healthier is a common but unpopular task for
most people who struggle with their weight.

But it can be done!

The real FAT facts:

· Obesity occurs as a result of having too much body fat.

· Everyone needs a certain amount of body fat to produce energy,
to manufacture hormones, insulate the body and provide shock
absorption.

· As a general rule, women carry more body fat than men.

- The World Health Organization suggests that men with more than 25 percent body fat and women with more than 30 percent body fat are obese.

- Obesity is associated with significantly increased risk of type 2 diabetes, hypertension, cardiovascular disease, certain forms of cancer, sleep apnea, and osteoarthritis.

- The current trend in obesity, and its health complications places a tremendous burden on our healthcare system and related costs.

Traditional approach

"In order to lose weight, you must count calories, keep track of everything you eat, and limit how much food you eat. Especially deprive yourself of the foods you most enjoy."

Most diets tell you exactly what food to eat and how much to eat, regardless of preferences or individual hunger pangs that you might experience. Although dieting can help you lose weight, it is often a short-term battle that is so unnatural and so unsustainable it never becomes a lifestyle you can maintain and enjoy.

"Dieting doesn't LAST"

Did you ever have this experience? Each time you quit the latest diet, you end up gaining back the weight you worked so hard to lose and sometimes even more!

Yo-yo dieting is detrimental to your health. Our attitudes and habits that we have developed through years of dieting have resulted in an obsession with body weight, poor self-esteem, improper nutrition and inappropriate exercise practices. Diets that are very strict usually result in temporary weight loss. However, their restrictions are so drastic that we cannot maintain them and they tend to drain us both physically and emotionally. In time, our old eating patterns reappear and serve another blow to our already low self-esteem. Unfortunately, most people who try to live by their food lists and rules learn very little or nothing at all about proper nutrition, healthy meal preparation, physical activity, or how to live a healthy lifestyle. One cannot live by dieting alone; we must commit to a lifestyle change to make this a lasting and enjoyable experience.

If your weight management program is to be successful, everything you eat, and every exercise you do, must be a pleasurable experience. If you are not enjoying yourself, you won't continue. It really is that simple. The small changes outlined in the Fit Family Program are not painful or overwhelming but are the core of an exciting lifestyle that you will look forward to every morning when you wake up!

This book gives you a method and lifestyle suggestions to help you stop dieting and start living the healthy lifestyle you have dreamed of.

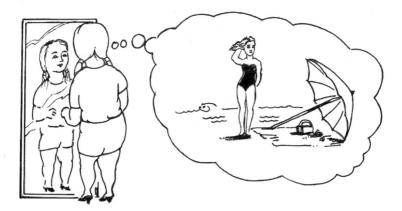

Eating too much? Burning too little? There's more to it than that.

They say it's a simple equation: obesity is the result of eating more calories than your body can burn. If only things were really this simple. Modern research has discovered that obesity is not caused by overeating alone. There are other factors that contribute to a person's ability to store fat. There are sound physiological reasons why some people can eat very large quantities of food and not increase their weight; while others seem to gain pounds from the mere smell of a rich, fatty treat! Hardly fair.

Genetic factors are passed down to us from our parents, and there are factors that we have brought on ourselves – improper hormonal balance, stress, poor food choices, and physical inactivity. Believe it or not, we have control over these factors and we can change how our body copes with them.

The naturopathic solutions proposed in this book include lifestyle modifications that will bring you success in personal weight loss, help you achieve optimum health for yourself and for those you love.

Beyond Dieting will teach you:
- the safest, most effective way to exercise
- how to deal with cravings
- how to overcome feelings of hunger
- ways to get your health and your family's health back on track.

Making it a family affair

I've developed the Fit Family Program to give individuals and families a more successful approach. Get the whole gang involved for more fun, and more incentive to stick with it.

The Fit Family Program offers methods and ideas on how to involve the whole family, or a group of friends, to help everyone towards their personal health and fitness goals.

With these tips you can actually create and control your environment so you will be successful. The program also addresses giving and getting positive reinforcement and rewards from family or group members to keep your motivation up and cheating down. You will learn how to create a team strategy and a sense of fun among the family, even if others don't share your specific health and weight loss goals.

"To eat is a necessity, but to eat intelligently is an art."
La Rochefoucauld

CHAPTER 1

My! How we've grown!

According to the New England Journal of Medicine, we are the first generation in history to be producing offspring with shorter life expectancies than our own. This devastating finding is a red alert that we must change our attitudes and habits if we want our children to enjoy better health and longer lives.

As a society we are falling victim to our own technological advancements. Microwaveable dinners, television as babysitter and sedative, and the oh-so-addictive, sit-and-stare internet. The level of physical activity among North Americans has declined dramatically over the past 50 years, and it shows in our state of health!

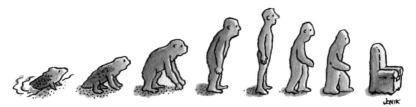

In 1960, the average 45 year old American woman weighed 143 pounds. (NHES 1: National Health Examination Survey, Cycle 1, Ages 20-74 years).

In 2002 the average weight of a 45 year old woman in the US was 168 pounds (NHANES: National Health and Nutrition Examination Survey).

Your grandmother might have walked a mile or two to get fresh fruits and vegetables three times per week, or she may have worked in the garden growing her own. Men and women walked to work, to school and even for pleasure and recreation (some still do). Other destinations? Well, email has certainly reduced trips to the post office. It can all be done from your desk.

And what about what we're putting in our mouths? We no longer cook fresh meats and vegetables on a regular basis. Check out the freezer. You'll find packaged meals that look like something they'd carry on a space shuttle! Convenience RULES! After all, we have to hurry back to the desk to check our email... I think you get the picture.

From Mammoth to Big Mac®: an historical look at food and fitness

Throughout history mankind has survived by finding food. Sometimes it's been difficult. Killing a mammoth was no small task. Foraging for berries and naturally available food, hunting anything that could be eaten, kept people moving from place to place to feed themselves and their families.

Droughts, famine, disease, wars, and financial devastation affected the availability of food, but humans have usually prevailed. One early survival datum was that the closer a food is to its original form (from the ground, tree, plant, or animal), the healthier it is for you. In other words, if native Americans ate fresh buffalo they were likely to be healthier than if they ate only smoked meat, one of the first types of "processed food". But animals could be infested with bacteria and disease, which were sometimes killed by cooking. With the introduction of industrialized farming, pesticides and environmental pollutants, the quality of our foods has declined.

The Industrial Age began mechanization of food production. For the first time in history food production and consumption increased due to the invention of both better machinery, which enabled more food output, and the evolution of transportation networks which carried food to the masses. For the first time food was coming to man rather than man having to go after his food. This was the turning point in history where food availability rose, while food quality declined.

In the 1900s to mid-1940s, most people remained fit and active out of necessity. Cars were not as affordable as they are today. The average person's daily pedometer reading would have been much higher than our are today. People worked in manual jobs which required good old elbow-grease to make a living – skilled trades, craftsmen, and farmers.

Without a refrigerator one could not keep foods cool enough to remain fresh for very long, so people went to the grocery store regularly. And lastly, processed food was rare; the daily diet contained more nutritious whole foods and very few additives and preservatives.

The 1950s and 60s brought in a new era of affordable automobiles, TV dinners and instant meals, full of preservatives and somewhat void of nutrients, which became part of the average family diet. Processing and preservation of food takes away a great deal of nutritional value. Even though man had landed on the moon, nutritional discoveries had not even taken off the ground. To some extent people stopped eating regular, sit-down meals – breakfast, lunch, dinner – and their physical activity also declined.

In the late 1970s we were introduced to the fast food restaurant. These were extremely "cool" and convenient, and they served foods high in delicious fats and starches, and low in vitamins, minerals and proteins. The fun factor of food was marketed to mothers and children very successfully. These restaurants have become a central focus in the lives of nearly every modern child or teen. Many adults find themselves eating with a steering wheel in front of them to save time, with potentially hazardous results, and not just for their waistlines!

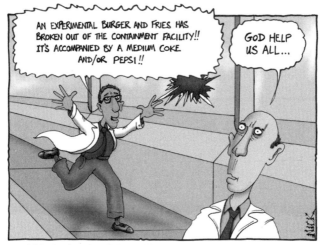

1964, the height of the cold war. In an average community surrounding a little-known biological warfare institute, the obesity epidemic is quietly unleashed.

From restaurants, to banking, and even our morning coffee, we have become a lazy society. We don't get out of our cars to perform even simple tasks. How many times have you waited in a drive-thru line for a coffee? How many times have you driven a few blocks to drop your child off at school?

Even our food is getting less exercise! The majority of North American cattle and farm animals are restricted to smaller and smaller pens and fields, so they move less. This can result in fattier cuts of meat.

Effort required to acquire food – DOWN

In the pre-agricultural age man had to hunt and gather his food; and this required a lot of physical effort. During the agricultural age man learned to farm and invented some equipment and machinery to harvest food. Yet this still required a lot of physical effort.

As man moved into the Industrial age he learned to build and harness machinery to do the work previously performed by man and beast, and as transportation improved less strenuous work was required to transport and exchange foods.

Today we can hop in the car or SUV and have food passed to us through the window, or simply pick up the telephone and order it! Compare the calories or energy used by our predecessors to acquire their food, and the amount of exercise we get today.

Daily exercise is a necessity for any weight loss program. According to IHRSA, statistics tell us that 13% of people in North America are a member of fitness club, but only 30% of members actually use it regularly. This translates into only 4% of our nation exercising regularly. This is a key factor in the weighty problems facing us.

Quality of food – DOWN

In the pre-agricultural age and the agricultural age everything that was eaten was from a natural source. Food sources may have had bugs but they were free of chemical pesticides and fertilizers, or genetic modifications. Today the majority of foods consumed by North Americans are not even fresh. They are pre-packaged, pre-cooked and they contain an array of additives and preservatives to keep them in an edible and presentable condition. Fresh fruits, vegetables and meats have all been subject to fertilizers, pesticides or feeds which enhance yields, but do little for nutritional value or flavour.

Frequency of food intake – DOWN

In the pre-agricultural age man simply ate whenever he had available food. Food was certainly not abundant and food could not be easily stored. Through the agricultural age man learned how to store certain types of food and whenever possible probably ate a standard 3 meals a day. The standard breakfast, lunch and dinner have remained with us in the western world into the1990s. Then as the workplace for many shifted from manual labour, which required regular food to be sustained, to more service industries, we started to see the average number of meals per day decline on the whole throughout the entire population.

The average American eats 2.5–2.7 meals per day (NHANES-III). Breakfast consumption habits have been linked to body weight, with breakfast skippers more likely to weigh more (Lin et al., 2004). On average, 55 percent of Americans reported eating breakfast. (NHANES-III)

The new "generation X"

Lack of physical activity is directly correlated to the functioning of your body's metabolism. The population is in a metabolic crisis right now and unless we step up and make a lifestyle change of our own, we will fall victim to the myriad of diseases that accompany unhealthy lifestyles. These diseases are preventable, treatable, and reversible.

You have metabolic syndrome if you have three of the following:

- ■ A waist greater than 40 inches for men, 35 inches for women
- ■ A triglyceride (blood fat) level of 150 mg/dL or higher
- ■ A "good" HDL cholesterol level of less than 40 mg/dL for men, less than 50 mg/dL for women
- ■ Systolic (the top number) blood pressure of 130 mm Hg or higher and diastolic (the bottom number) of 85 mm Hg or higher
- ■ A fasting glucose level of 110 mg/dL or higher – Insulin resistance (the body does not properly use insulin or blood sugar).

It is now estimated that Metabolic Syndrome affects approximately 47 million Americans (US Census Bureau, Population Estimates & International Data, 2004).

Source: National Cholesterol Education Program, ATP III Guidelines

What is the big deal with metabolic syndrome?

Metabolic syndrome is a serious disease because it is a red flag from our bodies that there is a serious disruption of physiological processes happening. There is a huge risk for suffering from potentially catastrophic health conditions with metabolic syndrome. You can think of it as a sign of the body in chaos, and CHAOS is a fitting acronym for complications that can arise from metabolic syndrome:

- **C**oronary artery disease
- **H**ypertension
- **A**dult onset diabetes
- **O**besity
- **S**troke

What causes metabolic syndrome?

Metabolic syndrome as well as type 2 diabetes, pre-diabetes, and obesity can all be viewed as different facets of the same disease having the same underlying dietary, lifestyle and genetic causes. The human body was simply not designed to handle the amount of refined sugar, salt, saturated fats, and other harmful food compounds that many people in Western countries consume, especially in those who live a sedentary lifestyle. The result is that a metabolic syndrome emerges with elevated insulin levels, obesity, elevated blood cholesterol and triglycerides, and high blood pressure.

Why today's diets are not working

The reason why 95% of all diets fail is simple. When you go on a low-calorie diet, your body believes that it is starving and it slows your metabolism down. Think of it as training your body to become more efficient at storing fat. Fat is a fuel source for your brain and your body is trying to conserve energy for your brain to function properly. When you stop this unrealistic eating regime, your metabolism is still slow and now more inefficient, causing your body to gain the weight back even faster, even though you may still be eating less than you were before you went on the diet.

You need muscle to maintain metabolic thermogenesis, the "burning" of fat for energy. Low-calorie diets cause you to lose both muscle and fat in relatively equal amounts. However, your rebound weight gain is all fat, not muscle, causing your metabolism to slow down even more. Now you are carrying extra weight, you have a less healthy body composition, and perhaps a less attractive physique. What can you do?

"One should eat to live, not live to eat."
Benjamin Franklin

CHAPTER 2

How to eat, what to eat, when to eat

There are a number of factors to consider when you begin a weight loss program; let's look them over and see how they relate to you.

What is the REAL cause of your weight gain?

For some people, the simple answer is, "I eat too much, and that is why I am overweight", however, it is rarely that simple. By applying certain naturopathic principles you can improve your weight as well as your overall health — and these changes can apply to the whole family. If you want to feel more energetic; if you want to lose weight and look better; the Beyond Dieting Fit Family program will help you and you can see your health improve!

Naturopathic principles of diet and nutrition

After treating hundreds of patients and counselling them on their weight loss goals, I have adapted the following core naturopathic principles:

1. Identify and treat the cause

The first principle of naturopathic medicine seeks to identify and to remove what may be causing your fatigue, lack of energy, and/ or weight gain. Rather than bombard you with temporary band-aid® solutions, it is necessary to get to the root of the problem. Since energy comes directly from the food and nutrients we provide ourselves with everyday, let's start there.

2. First do no harm

Naturopathic medicine follows three guidelines to minimize any discomfort for the patient:

· Using the least force or intervention necessary.

· Avoid, when possible, suppressing of symptoms.

· Acknowledge, respect and work with the individual's self-healing process.

3. Doctor as teacher

Naturopathic doctors share information and knowledge with their patients and encourage self- responsibility for health. As part of this program, it is very important to involve every member of your family in this healing process. You can take the responsibility to lead and teach these core values to other family members so that you can begin changing your lifestyle.

4. Treat the whole person

In naturopathic medicine we take into consideration the needs of each patient's physical, mental, emotional, genetic, environmental and social factors. This is also true for anyone attempting to change their lifestyle.

5. Emphasize prevention

Prevention is key. The average North American today is placing little emphasis on whole body, natural healing, but many want to and can do much to prevent further deterioriation of their health.

6. Support the healing power of the body

Our bodies have built-in self healing processes that are ordered and intelligent; respecting this phenomenon is an important step to achieving optimum health. Sometimes it is necessary to remove obstacles that prevent our own healing and recovery.

A healthy diet

The food you consume supplies your body with much more than energy to perform daily tasks. Food offers raw materials for all other body processes from keeping your bones strong, to strengthening your hair and nails. We need healthy food to strengthen our immune systems, improve our memory and mood, and to produce hormones. It is very important to eat the appropriate amount of fats, carbohydrates, and protein as well as making sure that you are getting the right amount of vitamins and minerals for your lifestyle. Remember, you are what you eat!

What do blood glucose and insulin have to do with weight loss?

The carbohydrates we eat are converted into one thing when they're digested: blood sugar, more accurately called glucose. It doesn't matter which type of carbohydrate you eat, a chocolate bar, a bowl of pasta, or a cup of broccoli, it's all converted into the same thing: glucose, blood sugar. Glucose is the basic fuel source used by all the cells in the body for energy. Your body is always trying to maintain a balanced blood sugar level to prevent hypoglycemia (low blood sugar) and hyperglycemia (high blood sugar).

Insulin is a hormone that responds directly to what you eat. Insulin is a major player in weight gain and it can actually keep you from losing weight. Insulin is responsible for the storage of energy from all the foods we eat: carbohydrates, proteins, and fats. Some carbohydrates cause blood sugars to rise suddenly, causing the pancreas to release insulin very rapidly and in some people the body overcompensates and releases far too much. The upside of this is you get a quick burst of energy; the downside is that most of what you've eaten will be stored as fat. Since blood sugars rose very rapidly, the insulin will try to bring blood sugar into a normal range very rapidly, causing the sugars to be pushed by the insulin into every cell, including fat cells. If, on the other hand, you eat certain other carbohydrates, blood sugar levels rise more slowly and so does insulin action. These have what is called a lower glycemic index (GI, see next section). When this happens, more of what you ate is pushed into your body's cells to be used for energy, and whatever is left over will be stored in fat cells.

By controlling the release of insulin with balanced meals, supplements and improved eating habits, you can control how much of your food turns to fat and how much is released for energy.

The glycemic index of foods

Any food that produces a rapid rise in blood sugar levels is called a high glycemic index (high GI) food. The glycemic index ranks carbohydrates based on the immediate effect they have on blood sugar levels. If your diet contains mostly high GI foods, your body is producing higher levels of insulin than if you were eating lower GI foods. If you have chronically elevated insulin levels your body is not simply converting blood sugar into energy, it is also storing extra "energy" in your body as fat. When insulin levels are high, you store more fat; when insulin levels are low, you burn fat more efficiently.

Choosing foods based on their Glycemic Index – the lower the GI, the better!

Choose Most Often Low Glycemic Index Foods	Choose Sometimes Medium Glycemic Index Foods	Choose Less Often High Glycemic Index Foods
Al dente (firm) pasta	Banana	Bagel, white
All-Bran™ cereal	Basmati rice	Cheerios™
Apples	Brown rice	Soda crackers
Carrots	Couscous	Digestive cookies
Chick peas	Pineapple	Dried dates
Grapes	Popcorn	French fries
Green peas	New potatoes	Ice cream
Lentils/kidney/baked beans	Raisins	Jellybeans
Oat bran bread	Rye bread	Parsnips
Oatmeal (slow cook oats)	Shredded wheat cereal	Potato, baked white
Oranges	Split or green pea soup	Potato, instant mashed
Peaches	Whole wheat bread	Rice, instant
Peanuts		Rice Krispies™
Pears		Rutabaga
Plums		Table sugar (sucrose)
Pumpernickel bread		Watermelon
Soy beverage		Whole wheat flour bread
Strawberries		White wheat flour bread
Sweet corn		
Sweet potato		
Plain Yogurt		

If you are consuming a diet that is rich in high GI foods, you probably experience cravings for carbohydrates and a ferocious appetite. The result? You will choose high GI foods and those foods will boost your insulin levels, producing a steady increase in weight. To stop this vicious cycle of overeating, we must address the metabolic syndrome you are experiencing – insulin resistance.

Insulin resistance and why you can't (couldn't) lose weight

Why can't you lose weight? One of the biggest reasons is because of the way your body handles glucose.If you overeat then your body produces more insulin. If this goes on for a long time you can become "insulin resistant", and your body metabolism will slow down, burning fewer of the calories you consume and "hanging on" to body fat. It is estimated 70 to 80 million Americans are resistant to the actions of insulin.

Almost all individuals with type 2 diabetes, and many with hypertension, cardiovascular disease, and obesity, are insulin resistant. People with insulin resistance tend to be overweight, often with lower levels of energy, mood swings, and increased muscle loss. It is well established that obesity leads to insulin insensitivity and vice versa. When fat cells, particularly those around the abdomen, become full of fat they secrete certain biological products that can dampen the effects of insulin, impair glucose utilization in muscles, and promote glucose production by the liver – more fat, less effective use of insulin. As the number and size of fat cells increase, they severely stress blood sugar control mechanisms and contribute to the development of the major complications of diabetes – atherosclerosis, nerve damage and blindness.

Insulin resistance and the "set point" theory

Research has found that each person has a programmed "set point" weight—the weight that a body tries to maintain by regulating its caloric intake. It has been thought that individual fat cells control this set point by sending out powerful messages to the brain to eat when they get smaller. Obese individuals have both more and larger fat cells, resulting in an overwhelming urge for them to eat.

The fact that this set point exists helps to explain why most diets don't work. While an obese or overweight person can fight off the urges to eat for a period of time, eventually these signals becomes too strong to ignore. This is one of the reasons why rebound overeating occurs and people often gain back all of their weight lost and more. This may result in re-setting their set point to a greater level. This is more commonly known as the "yo-yo" effect.

Understanding appetite

Appetite is a very complex urge that has evolved to help humans deal with food shortages. Unfortunately it is extremely biased towards weight gain. The desire to eat is a very sophisticated system that is supposed to tell the brain when the body requires more food as well as when to stop eating because enough food has been consumed. Most appetite-related signals originate in the gastrointestinal tract. Some hormones and compounds reduce appetite while others increase appetite. You would think you could just take an "appetite-suppressing" hormone, however, when an appetite suppressing hormone is given, the body responds with an increase in appetite stimulating compound!

Combatting insulin resistance

The benefits of soluble dietary fibre are well-known. Fibre helps the body lower cholesterol levels, improve blood sugar control, promote efficient elimination of waste, and reduce weight. The problem with dietary fibre supplements in the past has been that, in order to produce a true clinical effect, very large amounts of soluble fibre had to be consumed and a lot of gastrointestinal discomfort could result. A proprietary, highly viscous blend of glucomannan from konjac root, xanthum gum, and alginate, known as PGX® (PolyGlycopleX) has shown an ability to increase insulin sensitivity, and reduce factors that increase appetite while boosting those that decrease appetite.

When taken before meals, PGX® binds to water in the stomach and small intestine to form a gelatinous mass that provides a sense of fullness. In addition to reducing hunger and cravings, PGX® slows the absorption of sugars, and lowers cholesterol levels. It provides a higher level of viscosity and expansion with water than the same quantity of any other single fibre.

PGX® is the result of intense scientific research at the University of Toronto led by Vladimir Vuksan Ph.D., a recognized expert on the role of diet in diabetes, heart disease, and obesity. PGX® has the following benefits:

- Reduces postprandial (after-meal) blood glucose levels
- Increases insulin sensitivity
- Reduces appetite and promotes effective weight loss
- Improves diabetes control
- Lowers blood cholesterol

Handling blood sugar

Weight management, diabetes, pre-diabetes and metabolic syndrome are all health problems related to the body's ability to handle glucose. PGX® is a unique new way to help the body deal with blood sugar while supporting good nutrition and weight control.

Research Results: At the 64th Annual Meeting of the American Diabetes Association held in Orlando, Florida in 2004, the results of a clinical study using this proprietary fibre blend were presented by researchers from the Risk Factor Modification Centre at St. Michael's Hospital and the University of Toronto. Subjects with syndrome X took three grams of PGX® or placebo three times a day before meals. After three weeks, there was a 23% reduction in after-meal glucose levels, a 40% reduction in after meal insulin release, and a 55.9% improvement in the whole body insulin sensitivity scores. In addition, body fat was reduced by 2.8% from baseline following the 3-week period with this proprietary fibre blend.

Using PGX® to reduce and control weight

I have seen good results with the *No Nonsense Diet*® with PGX®. It is a powdered shake mix you can use to replace one or two meals a day. It also contains specific nutrients that help maintain healthy glycemic levels: Vitamin E (antioxidant), Vitamin C (antioxidant), Chromium (glucose tolerance factor), Zinc (supports the action of chromium), Magnesium (supports the action of chromium), Selenium (works synergistically with vitamin E). Another important ingredient in the *No Nonsense Diet*® shake mix is whey protein to support weight management. Increasing protein intake along with a low calorie diet and regular exercise has been shown to help promote both fat loss and healthy muscle growth.

Supplement recommendations

Losing and controlling weight can be different from person to person. Certain weight managment products offers tested, effective nutritional and herbal solutions for all the different aspects of weight loss. The following products offer a variety of ways to make your weight loss easier and more certain.

MetaSlim® Weight Reduction Formula with Bitter Orange extract, Yerba Mate extract, Green Tea extract, Cayenne Pepper, Ginger

These ingredients have been formulated to increase thermogenesis, in other words to stimulate the body to burn fat. Thermogenesis, as the name implies, is the generation of heat. Physical exercise is the best way to generate heat production in the body but even eating a meal causes a slight rise in body temperature. In the past, thermogenic weight loss formulas used ephedrine, a stimulating chemical, but it produced unwanted side effects in some people. MetaSlim® uses Bitter Orange (Citrus autantium), a member of the citrus orange family that supplies synephrine, a safer thermogenic stimulant for fat reduction. Synephrine occurs in virtually all citrus products. Citrus aurantium and other citrus species have long been used in Traditional Chinese Medicine.

MetaSlim® Weight Reduction Formula also contains caffeine, from Yerba mate and green tea extract, equivalent to less than one quarter cup of coffee per serving. Caffeine amplifies the thermogenic effects of synephrine. Yerba mate and green tea extracts have also been shown to facilitate weight reduction and are valued as herbal antioxidants. Several clinical studies have shown that increasing the intake of ginger and of cayenne pepper (Capsicum frutescens) increases fat burning.

CAUTIONS: If you are pregnant, lactating, taking MAO inhibitors or any other prescription drug medications, please consult with your physician before use.

MetaSlim® Carb Neutralizer & Fat Blocker, with Phaseolamin 2250 (Phase 2™), Cassia nomame extract and Gymnema sylvestre extract, is a natural non-stimulant product designed to do just what the name suggests – neutralize starch and block fat. It uses Phase2™, a mixture of compounds derived from white kidney beans, an ingredient clinically proven to neutralize the starch found in some of our favourite foods – potatoes, breads and pasta. Your body converts starchy carbohydrates into sugar. It does this by breaking-down the starch with the help of an enzyme (alpha amylase) produced in the pancreas. Phase2™ neutralizes the digestive enzyme alpha amylase before it can convert starch into glucose and then fat. Essentially, this formula allows starch to pass through the system undigested. Clinical and experimental studies indicate that Phase2™ can reduce digestion and absorption of about 85% of the starch eaten at a regular meal. This means you consume significantly fewer calories.

Cassia nomame is a member of the same family as cinnamon. It seems to contribute to weight loss by blocking lipase, the enzyme that digests fat, thereby reducing the amount of fat that is absorbed by your body when you eat (by up to 30 percent).

Gymnema sylvestre is a plant from India used in traditional medicine as a treatment for diabetes. Recent scientific investigation indicates that gymnema extract helps block the absorption of sugar as well as enhancing blood sugar regulation. This is important in curbing appetite and keeping the body burning fat between meals. Gymnema seems to improve the action of insulin and reduce cholesterol levels.

MetaSlim® Tonalin® CLA (conjugated linoleic acid) is a naturally occurring fatty acid that has been shown to reduce body fat and increase lean muscle mass. This is an essential fatty acid only obtained through our diet. CLA was primarily found in beef and dairy products and researchers believe we are getting much less CLA in our diets that in previous decades. Scientists are now able to produce CLA using the linoleic acid in natural safflower oil as well as sunflower oil, and converting it into conjugated linoleic acid. This is good news for vegetarians or those who have reduced their intake of meat and dairy. Studies have demonstrated that CLA inhibits the body's mechanism for storing fat; and can cause the body to utilize fatty reserve for energy. Results of human studies in Norway on CLA show that it helps individuals reduce body fat and promote lean muscle mass. These studies revealed no serious side effects from taking CLA.

Green Tea Extract is a common ingredient in many fat burners – it helps with thermogenesis and the metabolism of fat. It works without increasing the heart rate which is a concern with most fat burners. With green tea, dieters get the weight loss without the jitters and side effects. Green Tea contains a specific polyphenol, epigallocatechin gallate (EGCG) that appears to cause a reduction in food intake, and helps the body increase calorie and fat metabolism helping in weight management. Its weight loss effect may also be due to the caffeine content, which increases thermogenesis activity (increases fat and calorie burning) in the body.

The antioxidants in Green Tea may help decrease low-density lipoprotein (LDL) cholesterol and increase the levels of high-density lipoprotein (HDL), thus lowering "bad" cholesterol levels and increasing "good" ones. Cholesterol levels are an important factor in cardiovascular disease. Reported cancer prevention benefits of Green Tea would be due to its antioxidant content, which decreases the generation of free radicals.

MetaSlim® Fat Binding Fibre [NeOpuntia] is a nutritional supplement for weight management composed of fat binding dietary fibres, called NeOfibre and NeOmicel. These unique fibres attract and absorb the fat from foods and allow them to pass through the digestive system. The result is a reduction in the amount of fat that the body absorbs. Studies show NeOpuntia is a safe, natural choice to support weight loss.

*"You don't have to cook fancy or complicated masterpieces –
just good food from fresh ingredients."*
Julia Child

CHAPTER 3

Macronutrients – fats, carbohydrates, and protein

What is fat?

There was a time when we didn't know anything about fat except that it made foods tastier. We cooked with lard or shortening. We spread butter on our toast and we scooped sour cream onto our baked potatoes. However, since word got out that diets high in fat can increase our risk of heart disease, "no fat" and "low fat" have become the order of the day, but this doesn't have to be the case!

Eating a "low-fat" diet doesn't necessarily make one healthy. Look at the facts: in spite of the emphasis on low-fat diets and products people are fatter than ever before!

We need fat in our diet

Fat plays an essential role in our daily diets. Without dietary fat, we would not be able to absorb vitamins A, D, E, and K. Fat is digested slowly, staying in our intestines and keeping us satisfied longer after we eat. Fats are the most concentrated source of calories in our diet. They supply more than twice the number of calories per gram as carbohydrates or proteins.

Essential fatty acids, Omega-6 and Omega-3, are essential fats because our bodies cannot make them, we only get them through our diet. Saturated fats are the bad fats – they come from meat and dairy. The really bad saturated fat is called a trans fatty acid. Trans fats are processed fats that have been chemically altered and they are found in most packaged foods listed on the label as partially hydrogenated or hydrogenated oil. Our bodies prefer foods and oils in their natural (unprocessed) state.

Prosta WHATS?

Fats are converted in our bodies to what are called PROSTAGLAN-DINS. There are three types: PGE1, PGE2, and PGE3. Simply put, saturated fats (bad) convert into PGE2, which has an inflammatory effect on the body. Red meat is an example of a saturated fat and this is why patients who have had a heart attack are instructed to stay away from red meat! Omega-6 and Omega-3 fats are converted into PGE1 and PGE3 respectively and they produce an anti-inflammatory effect on the body. Good sources for essential Omega-3 fats are fish oils, seeds, particularly flaxseeds, nuts, leafy greens. Olive oil, and evening primrose oil are excellent sources of Omega-6.

All fats are not created equal

The fats we consume fall into one of three categories. These categories are:

· Saturated
· Monounsaturated
· Polyunsaturated

Saturated fats come from fatty cuts of meat, full fat milk and cheese, butter, cream, most processed baked goods such as cookies and pastries, most deep fried foods, coconut and palm oil. They are solid at room temperature. Eating a diet that is high in saturated fats can lead to elevated levels of 'bad' cholesterol (LDL) and put you at risk for other cardiovascular diseases. Experts agree that there exists a clear link between high blood cholesterol levels and heart disease.

Monounsaturated fats are found in foods such as peanuts, hazelnuts, cashews and almonds, avocadoes, and oils such as olive, canola and peanut oils. They help to raise the level of 'good' cholesterol (HDL) by helping the removal of cholesterol out of the blood.

Polyunsaturated fats come from fish oils, seafood, polyunsaturated margarines, vegetable oils such as safflower, sunflower, and corn or soy oils, nuts such as walnuts and Brazil nuts, and seeds. They are liquid at room temperature and must be stored in a cool, dark place because they react to light and temperature and break down rapidly.

Polyunsaturated fats can be divided into two categories:

- **Omega-3** fats are found in both plants and fish – they have been found to reduce the risk of heart disease.

- **Omega-6** fats are found primarily in nuts, seeds and plant oils such as corn, soy and safflower.

Dietary fats: Getting the right balance

Fats are very important for healthy development, but too much can cause health problems. For a healthy, well-balanced diet, it is recommended that you limit your calories from fat to 30 percent or less of your total calories. To make this even easier, here are some ways to cut back on saturated and polyunsaturated fats, while substituting some healthy monounsaturates:

- Choose leaner cuts of meat and trim the fat off before cooking.

- Replace meat with fish a couple of times a week. Steam, grill or poach fish – do not fry.

- Choose skinless chicken breast or turkey breast only.

- Drink skimmed milk, soy milk or rice milk

- Eat less cheese, and choose low-fat varieties.

- Eat low-fat yogurt and substitute it for cream and mayonnaise in cooking, dips and sauces.

- Eat well-balanced vegetarian meals rich in grains, legumes, and vegetables weekly.

- Use olive oil in salad dressings.

- Focus your meals around vegetables and grains and use meat as the "side dish" rather than the other way around.

The GOOD fats

These are fats that occur naturally and have not been damaged by high heat, refining, or processing. Good fats are found in fish, nuts, avocados, seeds and, believe it or not, butter.

Unfortunately, some of the best fats, such as flaxseed oil and fish oils, cannot be used for cooking because they respond badly to high heat. If you must cook with high heat, you're better off with something such as peanut oil, coconut oil or even lard, which are far more stable, yet not as healthy. I recommend cooking with low heat using olive oil or alternatively, fry using water and add the oil afterward – just to avoid heating the oil too much.

It is important to remember that the problem we have with fat is one of balance. We are simply not eating nearly enough omega-3s in proportion to other fats. Omega-3s are found in cold water fish, eggs, flaxseed oil and are available in supplement form.

Fat tips

Always include "good" fats in every meal. "Good" fats (known as monounsaturated fats) play an important role in the Fit Family Program. They can help balance blood sugar and control appetite. Sources of "good" fats include: olive oil, olives, avocado, almonds, macadamia nuts, and peanuts.

Avoid excess saturated fats. Try to limit your consumption of saturated fats to no more than 10% of your daily caloric intake.

Omega-3 versus Omega-6 – what's the story?

Just how do omega-3s perform so many health "miracles" in people? One way Omega-3 does this is by encouraging the production of body chemicals that help control inflammation in the joints, the bloodstream, and the tissues. Just as important is their ability to reduce any negative impact of yet another essential type of fatty acid known as omega-6s. Omega-6 is found in foods such as eggs, poultry, cereals, vegetable oils, baked goods, and margarine. Just like Omega-3, Omega-6s are also considered essential. They support skin health, lower cholesterol, and help make our blood 'sticky' so it is able to clot.

Problems occur in your body when Omega-6s aren't balanced with sufficient amounts of Omega-3s.

When your blood is too sticky it promotes clot formation and this can increase the risk of heart attacks and strokes. However, once you add Omega-3s to the mix, the risk of heart problems goes down.

The optimum ratio of essential fatty acids is roughly 4 parts Omega-3 to 1 part Omega-6. About an ounce (one handful) of walnuts has about 2.5 grams of Omega-3s, which is equal to about 3.5 ounces of salmon.

Supplement recommendations
Omega Oils

Lately people are hearing more and more about the health benefits of Omega-3, Omega-6 and Omega-9 fatty acids. Fatty acids are extremely important on our bodily metabolism regulation, brain development and function, circulation, hemoglobin production and immune function. They have a role in lowering blood cholesterol and pressure, contribute to healthy skin, hair and nails, and help relieve some symptoms of PMS, especially breast tenderness and uterine cramping.

Particularly important to good health are the longer chain omega-3 fatty acids such as eicosapentaenoic acid (EPA) and docosahexanoic acid (DHA) found in fish, especially cold-water fish such as salmon, mackerel, herring and halibut. EPA and DHA aid in reducing the 'bad' cholesterol (LDL cholesterol) and raise the 'good' HDL cholesterol. They also help lower blood fat, known as triglycerides, which if too elevated will present significant risk for heart disease. These Omega-3 polyunsaturated fatty acids are considered highly valuable as these are the forms the body requires most. These are some of the better ways to get sufficient and balanced amounts of healthy Omega oils.

Webber naturals™ Omega 3 Super Concentrate [EPA 400 DHA 200]
Unique Canadian processed Super Concentrate Omega-3 Oil. This pharmaceutical grade product has the highest levels of EPA & DHA on the market. Many consumers feel they need only Omega-3 and get enough Omega-6 and 9 through a typical North American diet. Most heart attacks are precipitated "out of the blue" because an inappropri-

ate blood clot wedges itself into a coronary artery in the heart, effectively ending blood flow to a critical segment of the heart muscle, causing it to die. EPA and DHA significantly reduce the risk of inappropriate blood clotting which can also lead to stroke or pulmonary embolism, as life threatening as a heart attack.

Webber naturals™ Omega 3-6-9 Extra Strength (High Lignan)

Omega fatty acids are important for overall health and well being from the inside out! Essential fatty acids are only obtained through our diets, however most North Americans are lacking in these good fats.

Balanced omega 3-6-9 oils can help:

- Improve skin conditions like eczema and dull hair
- Help relieve digestive disorders
- Support brain function and development
- Improve blood pressure and lower cholesterol and triglyceride levels
- Relieve PMS and uterine cramping
- Oils are cold pressed, solvent free and protected in dark coloured softgels

Each softgel capsule contains: Flaxseed Oil 400 mg, Fish Oil blend (180:120) 400 mg, Borage Oil 400 mg

*Lignans are natural phytochemicals found in high concentrations in flaxseeds and in this unique oil.

Webber naturals™ Salmon & Fish Oil 1000mg 180:120

Webber naturals™ Salmon Oil is a superior source of Omega-3 fatty acids, particularly eicosapentaenoic acid (EPA) and docosahexaenoic acid (DHA). Webber naturals™ 1000 mg product supplies 180 mg of EPA and 120 mg of DHA per capsule.

Fish oils help keep blood thin and reduce the risk of clots, so persons on blood thinning medication should check with their nutritionally-oriented doctor before taking them. Fish oils are not recommended for people with a tendency to hemorrhage or who have bleeding disorders, such as hemophilia. Anyone taking fish oil supplements should also take 200 to 400 IU of natural-source vitamin E to prevent the formation of damaging free radicals that result when the body metabolizes the oil.

What are carbohydrates?

Carbohydrates exist in a wide variety of foods – bread, beans, milk, popcorn, potatoes, cookies, spaghetti, corn, and candy. The most common and abundant forms of carbohydrates are sugars, fibres, and starches. The basic building blocks of carbohydrates are sugars – which are found in virtually all plant-based food sources.

Examples are: grains (the basis of all pastas, breads, and cereals), fruits, vegetables, beans, rice, and potatoes.

As discussed earlier in this chapter, carbohydrates are classified based on the glycemic index, which measures how fast and how far blood sugar rises after you eat a food that contains carbohydrates. For example, when you eat white rice, it is almost immediately converted to blood sugar, causing a rapid spike in both blood sugar and insulin. Therefore, it is classified as having a high glycemic index. Brown rice on the other hand is digested more slowly, causing a lower and gentler change in blood sugar – it has a low glycemic index. Due to the potentially negative effects that different types of carbohydrates can have on your health, it is essential to healthy eating to choose the right carbohydrates.

Now, this does not mean that you should avoid all carbohydrates. Carbohydrates are very important for the proper functioning of your body. Nature makes plenty of healthy carbohydrates that are beneficial – fruits, vegetables, beans, lentils, whole grains – strive to choose these options in your diet.

What is protein?

Protein is an essential nutrient for cell maintenance and repair, as well as regulation of a wide range of bodily functions. You need protein to make enzymes and hormones that are necessary for proper digestion, metabolism, and tissue growth and repair. How much protein we need to eat in our diet usually depends on our lean muscle mass and level of physical activity.

The best sources of protein come from animal products – eggs, milk, and meat. However, protein is found in all meats and vegetables. Certain vegetable proteins can be eaten together to form a complete protein for proper amino-acid ratios. If you are a vegetarian, it is important to pay close attention to eating the proper combinations of protein-rich vegetables.

Aim for high quality proteins at every meal. By including a low-fat, high quality protein at each meal, you can help stimulate the release of glucagon, which is a mobilization hormone. Glucagon keeps blood sugar balanced to maintain peak mental focus. Meats that I affectionately deem "mystery meats" like luncheon slices, Spam®, and hot dogs, should be avoided as they do not offer much nutritive value. Some examples of low-fat, high-quality proteins are: chicken, turkey, fish, lean cuts of beef, egg whites, tofu, beans and cottage cheese.

Protein basics

The following information should provide some understanding of daily protein requirements and how to use protein supplements. Most athletes who use protein supplementation choose whey protein. Even though these notes reflect a largely athletic perspective, daily hard manual work also requires protein for energy and strength.

1. Intense exercise causes cannibalization of muscle protein for energy and repair to micro injuries as they occur. Some protein is also lost in the urine, resulting in an overall net loss of body protein.

2. Replacing this protein through the diet, helps maintain your muscle size and strength.

3. Regular strenuous exercise (work) requires more than 0.80 grams per kilogram per day to maintain muscle mass. Approximately 1.4 to 1.8 grams of protein per kilogram of body weight is needed to maintain muscle mass in athletes involved in endurance exercise like running, cycling and swimming. Most meats contain approximately 25% actual protein. Eating only meat as a protein source may present practical problems and that is why protein drinks are so popular with athletes, and with busy active people.

4. New muscle mass growth occurs in proportion to the level of exercise imposed on a muscle. Merely eating more protein will not cause muscle growth.

Use of protein supplements should be based on the amount of protein required to meet your daily protein intake RDA. The table below shows guidelines.

Recommended Daily Intakes of High-Quality Protein Under Normal Conditions

Age (years)	Reference Weight (Kg)	RDA (g/kg/day)
0-0.5	6	2.2
0.5-1	9	1.6
1-3	13	1.2
4-6	20	1.1
7-10	28	1.0
11-14 males	45	1.0
11-14 females	46	1.0
15-18 males	66	0.9
15-18 females	55	0.8
19+ males	72-79	0.8
19+ females	58-65	0.8

During pregnancy, add 10 grams per day
Lactation, first 6 months, add 15 grams per day
Lactation, second 6 months, add 12 grams per day

Food and Nutrition Board, National Research Council, Recommended Dietary Allowances, 10th edition, Washington, DC, National Academy Press, 1989. Adapted from reference.

Whey protein

Whey protein is the most popular choice of protein for athletes. Extra protein consumption is necessary for anyone doing serious training or competition if they want to avoid muscle mass loss due to wasting, and to build new muscle. A good brand of whey product will be produced using "cross-flow micro-filtration" and will be high quality low fat and low lactose.

Because whey protein products have a high percent of actual protein, whey supplementation gives you better control over the amount of protein you consume.

A very important part of sport nutrition is the support of tissue repair, particularly connective tissue like tendons, ligaments and the fibrous tissue that encases muscle fibres into working bundles. All connective tissue repairs are driven by glucosamine, which is completely dependent on available glutamine for its production. Whey protein contributes to the production of glutamine and glucosamine, so it is important to connective tissue repair. A good whey protein will also contain bromelain, a pineapple enzyme that helps digest the protein and helps to reduce swelling and inflammation and promote wound healing.

The best times to consume whey protein are right after exercise, one hour before meals, 40 minutes before exercise, before bed, and first thing in the morning. Consume whey protein on an empty stomach for rapid absorption.

Soy and other proteins

Soy protein is a complete protein, meaning that it provides all the essential amino acids needed to fulfill the human nutritional requirements for growth, maintenance, physical stress, and general health for children and adults. Soy protein can be used as the sole protein source, but is complemented by other proteins found in grains, legumes, and other plants, as well as by animal protein choices.

Regular consumption of soy protein for nutrition reasons, is also associated with key health benefits created by two isoflavones, called genistein and daidzein, plant estrogen-like compounds naturally present in soybeans. Consuming as little as 25 grams daily of soy protein, as part of a reduced fat diet, supplies enough soy isoflavones to have a significant cholesterol lowering effect on the total cholesterol, the LDL cholesterol, and triglycerides, while significantly raising HDL.

As well, studies indicate that isoflavones have a protective effect against breast, prostate, and colon cancers. The versatile isoflavones, acting as weak estrogens, have been shown to have a positive effect on bone mineral density, and to improve the quality of life for many postmenopausal women, especially reducing the intensity and frequency of hot flashes. Population studies with Asian women, who normally consume high amounts of soy isoflavones, suggest that soy is protective against breast cancer. However, some researchers believe isoflavones could actually exert an unwanted estrogenic affect and increase the risk of breast cancer.

Beans, chick peas, lentils, nuts and seeds are excellent sources of protein and have the added benefit of containing fibre, vitamins and minerals, especially when combined with whole grains such as millet, buckwheat and brown rice. Vegetable-based proteins are low in fat, high in fibre, inexpensive and readily available, and they contain numerous phytochemicals (chemicals found in plants) that contribute towards health and disease prevention.

Complimentary Proteins

Combine one choice from each list to make a complete protein.

Kidney Beans	Bread
White Beans	Pasta
Lima Beans	Rice
Lentils	Bulgur
Chick Peas	Couscous
Green Peas	Corn
Black-eyed Peas	Almonds
Peanuts	Sesame Seeds

Fibre

Dietary fibre plays an important role in providing support to your gastrointestinal system. Poor colon health can lead to constipation, hemorrhoids, colitis, and chronic fatigue. Fibre in your diet slows the rate of digestion, which helps promote a more steady release of insulin and blood sugar following a meal. Added benefits of fibre include a sense of fullness following a meal which reduces your appetite. Good sources of fibre include bran, beans, brown rice, and green vegetables. A powdered fibre supplement such as PGX®, can also be used to ensure an adequate daily fibre intake as well as to improve your body's utilization of blood sugar and to reverse insulin resistance. Daily fibre intake should match or exceed the RDA of 25-35 grams. (For more information on PGX®, see chapter 2, page 19.)

Water

Water plays a very important role in how well our body functions. Aside from 60–70% of your body being composed of water, life and health depend highly on those two hydrogen and one oxygen molecules. Water assists digestion with absorption and assimilation of food; it assists in excretion of waste from the bowel and kidneys; it regulates body temperature and, since your blood is 92% water, it is an integral part of your body's transport system, distributing nutrients around the body.

Water is a natural appetite suppressant. Lack of water can lead to over eating because your brain does not differentiate between hunger and thirst. Often, when you think you are hungry your body may in fact be signaling that you are thirsty! In many instances people find what they thought were hunger pangs were in fact, satisfied by water. Try it! You have nothing to lose, except some weight.

How do you know how much water to drink each day? It is best to drink at least one half of your body weight in ounces. For example, if you are a 150 pound person, you need to drink 75 ounces. The goal is to drink water consistently throughout the day, rather than all at once. If you drink an abundance of caffeinated beverages, you are drinking diuretics! They cause your body to naturally lose water and thus you should drink one extra glass of water for every caffeinated beverage you consume each day.

Tips to increase your water intake – drink throughout the day!

In the morning when you wake up you will often be thirsty because your body loses water while you are sleeping through breathing and perspiration. Drink a large glass of water immediately upon waking and add a slice of lemon if you wish for flavour.

- **Breakfast:** Drink another glass of water with breakfast or substitute with a cup of herbal tea.

- **Mid morning:** Snack on a piece of juicy fruit and have another glass of water. Perhaps add some chlorella or spirulina for added health benefits.

- **Lunch:** Have some soup for lunch or have a glass of water or herbal tea before your meal.

- **Mid afternoon:** Snack on some crunchy vegetables and drink a glass of water while you are preparing your evening meal.

- **Dinner:** Drink a glass of water before your meal with 1-2 tsp of apple cider vinegar to improve your digestion.

- **Evening:** Before going to bed, drink your final glass of water and retire for the night!

When you start to increase your daily water intake, there are many great benefits. You may notice your skin tone significantly improve and even better recovery in your muscles. Many people find that they have increased energy, and decreased constipation and headaches, as well as reduced hunger pains.

Signs that you may be dehydrated

- **Headaches.** Your brain is 75% water, so even slight dehydration can cause headaches.

- **Poor concentration and fatigue.** Lack of water is a major cause of daytime fatigue. Water is essential in flushing toxins from the body. If you cannot eliminate toxins, you will have less energy as your body tries to cope with the added toxins and stress.

- **Constipation.** When you are dehydrated, your body chooses to use water where it is needed in order of importance – away from your bowels, resulting in hard, dry stools which are difficult to expel.

- **Deep-coloured urine or lack of urination.**

- **Bad breath.** Water washes away food particles from your mouth – leaving less for the bacteria to grow on.

- **Dry, non-elastic skin.** Pinch the skin on top of your hand. If it doesn't snap back immediately like an elastic, you may be dehydrated.

- **Dry Eyes, Mouth, or nasal passages.**

"As a child my family's menu consisted of
two choices: take it or leave it."
Buddy Hackett

CHAPTER 4

Fit Family Program

The food that you consume supplies your body with much more than
energy to perform daily tasks. Food offers raw materials for all other
body processes, from keeping your bones strong, to strengthening
your hair and nails. We need to "feed" our immune systems, our
memory and mood, and our hormones. It is very important to eat the
right balance of fats, carbohydrates, and protein, as well as using vitamin and mineral supplements to support your lifestyle.

If you are reading this book then you want to lose weight and/or
become healthier. You may have tried to improve your weight and
health before with limited success. Read this chapter carefully – it will
help you succeed this time around.

The Fit Family Program is based on concepts and ideas adapted from
the works of James O. Prochaska, John C. Norcross and Carlo
DiClemente, three PhD researchers who have conducted years of clinical studies on behavioral change.

Six stages of change

There are six stages you go through in order to achieve any lifestyle
change. No one stage is any more important than the other. To be
successful you must go through each of the six stages.

1. **Pre-contemplation:** Not quite thinking about it yet. People at the
   pre-contemplation stage do not recognize that they have a problem
   with a specific behavior and they have no intention of changing.
   Pre-contemplators would rather change those around them than
   change themselves.

2. **Contemplation:** Starting to think about it. In this stage people recognize that they have a problem and start to think about ways of solving it. They see causes and think about possible solutions. Contemplators may be far from taking any action and they have indefinite plans, "maybe I'll do something within the next 6 months".

3. **Preparation:** Now I've got to do something about this. People at the preparation stage are close to making a decision, close to taking some action towards solving their problem, but they can still be up to 2 months away from actually starting.

4. **Action:** I'm doing it now! The action stage is where people start to modify their problematic behavior. Of course this stage requires the most commitment. Most people think the action stage IS the change rather than identifying it as just one of the stages required to be successful.

5. **Maintenance:** Keep it going! The maintenance stage is where new behaviors are learned and consolidated. Maintenance requires effort in terms of keeping up the new behavior and avoiding falling back into old behaviors. This stage can last as little as 6 months or as long as a lifetime.

6. **Termination:** I'm done! This stage is where the person has succeeded in adopting a new behavior pattern and has been achieved a goal. There is no reverting to old habits.

Relapse

There is also one more stage, which is relapse. Someone may have advanced toward their goal, but has then fallen back to a former stage.

This is a basic overview of the different stages that people go through in order to achieve successful change. As you can see each stage has different life spans and within each stage people can benefit from different kinds of help and techniques in order to progress them to the next stage. Change can be achieved short term through different methods but in order to be truly successful a person will need to go through each stage.

Preparing to change your life

Unfortunately when it comes to weight loss, or trying to lead a healthier life, most people are destined to fail before they begin. This can be due to a lack of preparation and planning. To ensure long-term success time must be spent in the planning phase. Take some time to sit back, plan, and put into place all the things that will lead to your success. In this chapter we discuss some successful planning steps you can take to ensure you make it to your goal.

Set goals

Make a list of the benefits you will experience when you have achieved your weight loss and lifestyle targets. Post these benefits in several prominent places around the house where you will see them throughout each day. Top spots are: the fridge door, the back of the bathroom door and on the mirror you look into every morning. This will remind you of your end goal and the long-term benefits, and will help you overcome the desire to fall back into old habits.

Once your goals are set, and clear in your mind, then measure yourself against those goals on an ongoing basis, and be sure to reward yourself when you succeed! I suggest you measure yourself against your goals as frequently as possible to ensure that you stay focused. If you do not measure yourself against your goals regularly enough you will not get the feedback needed to adjust your plan. Imagine you were building a wall made of bricks and you wanted this wall to be level and straight. The best way to ensure it ends up being straight is to measure after you lay each brick with a level. If you do not measure until half the wall is done and it is not level there is a temptation to stop building the wall or quit completely. Constant feedback keeps you focused and allows you to make the necessary adjustments along the way.

Rewards count!

Rewards aren't necessarily food "treats". In fact, avoid using things you are trying to avoid as rewards. Make your rewards small and frequent. Also, decide on a very large reward, the largest most expensive most outrageous reward you can afford, to help you keep your eye on your final goal!

Write it down

Start by writing down your goal. This could be a number of pounds you wish to lose, a new pant size, a blood pressure level, or a cholesterol level, or the number of miles you wish to be able to run. MAKE IT MEASUREABLE. Your goals need to be specific and measurable. Take small steps as you begin and be ready with the resources you need when you start. Substitute a few healthy food choices for your less than healthy ones. Substitute one good meal or snack for one "bad" one each day or every other day to start.

Environment control

How's your space? If I were to come to your house right now and take a food audit, how many temptation foods would I find? How many bags of chips, boxes of cookies or chocolate bars? How many sweet or fatty treats are in your space that could stand in the way of you achieving your weight loss goals? Remember, if it isn't there you can't eat it. Set yourself up for success; make it easier not to fail by cleansing your house of all and any foods which are not going to be part of the new you and your new family lifestyle.

How many times per week do you put yourself in places where it is hard to control your food intake? Where do you eat lunch everyday and with whom? Are you visiting fast food restaurants with others? Eliminate "environmental temptation" created by the coffee shop, the bakery, the fast food place, even the convenience store.

Try the following:

- Eat lunch daily with someone who also wants to lose weight and eat well.

- Avoid placing yourself in environments where you will be tempted.

- When you feel temptation call a friend and get support or take a walk.

- Rid your house of all foods that don't reflect your new approach to nutrition.

Set the date

Setting a definite date to start is critical. This stops further procrastination and can also ensure that you do not start too soon without sufficient preparation. Once you have the date, don't delay or find excuses to change it. You want a date that will give you a good start without any interruptions, like special occasions or holidays.

Make an announcement

This is probably one of the hardest steps. Get moral support by creating a network of people who can help you succeed. Tell these people about your plans and goal. Most people skip this critical step and because they are worried that they may fail and will then feel even worse. By telling others about your plans you can enlist their support and they can help you get there.

The Fit Family Weight Loss Meeting

Who, besides YOU, has the most to do with what you eat? Most people would say "the family". Whether you are trying to lose weight alone or as a family, a team approach can be successful. Each family member has a role to play if everyone is to achieve their goals.

STEP 1: Hold a family meeting.

Who's in and who's not?

You will need to find out from each adult family member which of them is 100% committed to making a lifestyle change. There is no point trying to force anyone to go forward with the new plan unless they have bought into the plan and want to make a change. It is okay if certain family members do not want to make a change at this stage, however they will need to play role in supporting those who wish to make changes.

STEP 2: Each family member names their goal.

See the goal setting section in the previous chapter.

STEP 3: Each decides how they can help the others and how the others can help them.

Once you have established who is going to follow the new plan and who is not, you will need to clearly communicate why this is important to each of you and what the benefits will be. You need to be specific and detailed here so that everyone can see why this new lifestyle will eventually benefit them. For example a mother may explain to her teenage daughter that she feels she wants to lose weight so that she will be at less risk of disease in the future, look and feel better about herself and also be able to participate in more activities in the future with her family.

Suggestions

- Make a list of "banned foods" – No banned foods are to be brought into the house.

- Banned foods will only be permitted into the home environment once a week and will not remain in the home for more than 24 hours.

- Banned foods will be permitted into the house but will be locked away in a specific area. Access will only be given to those who are not partaking in the weight loss plan. In addition those who are not on the weight loss plan agree not to access the locked area and flaunt banned foods in front of others.

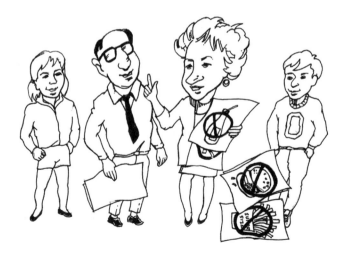

Priorities

To be successful your weight loss or new healthy lifestyle needs to be moved up your priority list in life. This is like preparing for an operation. Prepare those around you for how you may change before during and after you start. You may have more energy, decreased mood swings, increased self-esteem, and perhaps even disease symptoms will disappear! You need to be aware of these and let friends and family know so they can support you and cheer you on.

The more you know about nutrition and exercise and the effects on your body, the more likely you are to succeed. For example, many women put on extra weight after they have started to exercise using weights because "muscle weighs more than fat" and weight training can reduce body fat percentage. Knowing this can help you avoid disappointment. Focus on how you look and fit into your clothes.

Create your plan of attack

Are you going to go for a drastic change or are you going to take a slower approach and slowly wean yourself into your new habits? Each can be successful and both will work for different types of people however to be successful you will need to have taken the appropriate measures in planning for your given strategy.

You will also need to keep track of your progress DAILY in detail so you can measure how you are doing against your plan. If you plan to wean yourself out of your old habits and into your new ones, what are the criteria you will use to measure your success as you go along? Carry a notebook and a pen. Writing down what you eat and drink forces an awareness of what you are putting into your body.

At the end of each month see how you've progressed and set new goals. If you did not achieve your goals, don't quit. Simply revaluate and carry on.

10 weight loss essentials

Although you have set your goals and are committed to losing weight, there still seem to be barriers in your way. Good nutrition alone will not make you lose weight, you must also alter other aspects of your lifestyle – sleep, stress, and even mood. Neglecting any of these is like throwing a wrench into your entire program.

1. **Sleep.** Do not cheat yourself of a good night's rest. If you deprive your body of sleep, it must find energy in other ways, meaning eating more calories to stay awake and alert. Also, when we are tired, we tend to make poorer food choices and will eat foods that give us immediate pleasure. Enough sleep is important, but regulate yourself with an alarm clock. Try to go to sleep and wake at the same times each day (within reason). Ideally you should be in bed by 11:00pm and awake by 7:00am. This will help to regulate your circadian rhythms (your sleep-wake cycle) and has a profound effect on mood regulation.

2. **Combination of Diet and Exercise.** Without combining these two elements your success will be limited. A lot of people think that because they exercise, they can eat whatever they want – but this is not the case. Working out will help to gain muscle, but unless they cut back on calories, they may not notice a change in their actual size. A regular exercise schedule which includes both cardio and strength training is a very important part of your program. You must be active and try to do some exercise every day, even if it is just doing some yoga and/or stretching in front of the TV at night.

3. **Stress Management.** When you're stressed out, your body is lacking in a number of areas – sleep, nutrition, digestion, and overall sense of well-being. Similar to sleep deprivation, when people are under stress, they reach for food to cope. When someone's life is filled with stress, they feel like time is limited and neglect exercise even though it is one of the best things you can do to lower your stress level.

4. **Don't Skip Meals.** Skipping meals will play havoc with your blood sugar levels and will program your body to store additional fat. You may also lower your metabolic rate and lose muscle tis-

sue. Your body goes into starvation mode and your metabolism becomes sluggish to compensate for the lack of fuel. Instead of missing a meal, use a nutrition bar or meal replacement powder to make a nutritious drink. These can help you stick to your program when you don't have the time for a "sit-down" meal. People who eat breakfast everyday consume fewer total calories during the day then those who don't.

5. **Avoid Late Night Eating.** Eat dinner no less than 4 hours before bedtime. For example, if you regularly go to bed at 11 pm, do not eat dinner after 7 pm. Snacks are allowed 3 hours before bed. Try to not eat past 8pm. Your body begins to slow down its metabolic rate in the evening as it prepares for the overnight fast and repair processes that occur while you sleep.

6. **Don't be Discouraged.** Aim for consistency in your lifestyle, not perfection. You will have the occasional meal that's not perfect. When you get off track, don't let it slow you down! Make it positive and enjoy the divergence; then rekindle your goals and get back on your program with your very next meal.

7. **Control Calories.** Try not to consume more than 500 calories per meal for males and 400 calories per meal for females. This is the maximum number of calories most people can consume and metabolize in one meal without storing fat. Never eat until you are over-full. Notice the feeling of fullness and stop eating! Also notice when you get hungry.

8. **Learn Portion Control.** Use these guidelines:

   · Your portion of protein should not exceed the size and thickness of your palm;

   · Your fruits and vegetables (excluding calorie-dense starches) should equal that of two loose fists.

   · If you are eating a high-glycemic starchy carbohydrate (potatoes, pasta, white rice, or breads), your portion should equal the size of one clenched fist.

9. **Water Intake.** It is not uncommon to mistake hunger for thirst. Keeping yourself well hydrated during the day will discourage this misjudgement.

10. **Use Supplements for Support.** There are many natural products that can help you control your appetite, burn fat and improve metabolism so losing weight becomes easier. Review the product lists at the end of each chapter and see if some of these products are right for you.

*"Children are one third of our population
and all of our future."*
Panel for the Promotion of Child Health, 1981

CHAPTER 5

Raising healthy children in a fast food world

There are an increasing number of children who are overweight, and if no intervention is made, many of them will become overweight adults. This lifestyle puts them at risk for many medical problems, including diabetes, high blood pressure, high cholesterol, and sleep apnea. As well, obesity can adversely affect their self esteem.

All children, like adults, normally need a certain number of calories each day that their bodies use as energy for normal daily activities (walking, breathing, etc.). This ranges for boys from 2000 calories for a 7-10 year old, 2500 calories for an 11-14 year old, and 3000 calories for a 15-18 year old. For girls the ranges are from 2000 calories for a 7-10 year old, to 2200 calories for an 11-18 year old. These are only estimates and some children need more (fast metabolism) or less (slow metabolism) of an energy allowance for daily activities.

The same principles apply to children as to adults. If a child consumes more food and calories than they are burning in a day, then those excess calories are converted to fat for storage. Conversely, if a child consumes less food and calories than they are burning in a day, then their body fat is converted to energy for the needed calories.

While it is not healthy to put your child on a severely restricted diet, you should encourage weight management with a combined approach of a sensible diet and regular exercise.

Our culture with its emphasis on quick, comfort foods has had a negative impact on the health of our children. According to the New England Journal of Medicine, January 2005, we are the first generation in human history to be producing offspring with shorter life expectancies than our own. We can attribute much of this finding to the lifestyle that we are cultivating and passing down to our children. Do not depend on physical education classes at school, since we know there have been changes to the elementary school curriculum since we were students. It is more important than ever to get our children off the couch and into more physical activities.

Motivate your child

It will be much easier for your child to lose weight there is a drive to achieve this goal. You can help your child to lose weight by making healthy choices for his meals at home and encouraging regular exercise and physical activity.

Try to include your child in the process of eating healthier and exercising regularly. Bring them to the grocery store with you and teach them how to prepare simple, yet healthy snacks and meals. It may also help to use praise and simple rewards when your child is eating well and is being physically active. It is very important to avoid and negative talk or putting your child down when they are not motivated.

Set realistic goals with your child

First things first. Your first goal in weight management in children should be to stop weight gain and maintain normal growth in height. It's important to emphasize that the focus needs to be in growing (height) into their weight. To do this, begin by having your child eat healthier (about 500 fewer calories each day) and begin a program of regular exercise and physical activity.

Once your child has stopped gaining weight and is on a regular program of dieting and exercising, you can set further goals of slow weight loss (about a 10% reduction at a time) if necessary.

Modify behavior

It is important to modify the behaviors that led your child to become overweight and prevent weight loss, including:

· **Replace Spectating with Action:** Limit television viewing, including playing video games or using the computer, to about one or two hours each day; Children need exercise (even if disguised as playing!) to grow up strong and healthy. A body that gets exercise will also have an appetite for healthier foods.

· **Healthy Eating Habits:** Your child should eat three well-balanced meals of average size each day, plus two nutritious snacks. Breakfast is essential!

· **Snacks:** Limited to two per day, snacks can be low-calorie, such as raw fruits or vegetables. Avoid high calorie or high fat foods for snacks, especially chips, cookies, etc.

· **Drinking:** Encourage your child to drink four to six glasses of water each day, especially before meals. Water has no calories and it will help you to feel full. Avoid letting your child drink soft drinks or fruit juices, as they are high in calories and sugar.

· **Diet Diary:** Help your child keep a weekly journal of food and beverage intake and also of the amount of time spent watching television, playing video games and exercising.

Lead by example

Children learn by example and who best to set the example than the ones they love the most – their parents. Help yourself and your child by becoming more educated about the foods you eat, how many calories they contain, and where these calories come from.

Learn to read food labels

When you are reading the nutrition facts on a food label, start at the top. The most important things are listed from top to bottom.

Serving size

It is important to pay close attention to the serving size and to be aware of how many servings you are consuming. Sometimes the number of servings in the package is double or triple what is on the nutrition facts, therefore eating the whole package means you would have to double or increase the caloric intake. A "serving" of potato chips might only have 200 calories, but maybe the serving size is only 10 chips. Eating the whole bag could equal more than 1000 calories!

Percent Daily Value

Nutrition Facts
Serving Size 2 crackers (14 g)
Servings Per Container About 21

Amount Per Serving	
Calories 60	Calories from Fat 15

	% Daily Value*
Total Fat 1.5g	**2%**
Saturated Fat 0g	**0%**
Trans Fat 0g	
Cholesterol 0mg	**0%**
Sodium 70mg	**3%**
Total Carbohydrate 10g	**3%**
Dietary Fiber Less than 1g	**3%**
Sugars 0g	
Protein 2g	

Vitamin A 0%	•	Vitamin C 0%
Calcium 0%	•	Iron 2%

* Percent Daily Values are based on a 2,000 calorie diet. Your daily values may be higher or lower depending on your calorie needs:

		Calories:	2,000	2,500
Total Fat	Less than		66g	90g
Sat Fat	Less than		20g	25g
Cholesterol	Less than		300mg	300mg
Sodium	Less than		2400mg	2400mg
Total Carbohydrate			300g	375g
Dietary Fiber			25g	30g

The percentages that you see on food labels are based on recommended daily allowances – meaning the amount of something a person should get each day to prevent nutrient deficiency diseases. For instance, there's a recommended daily allowance for fat, so the food label might say that one serving of this food meets 10% of the daily value. Daily values are based on the needs of an adult, not a child. The needs of a child are often similar, but children may need more or less of certain nutrients, depending on their age and size.

Some percent daily values are based on the amount of calories and energy a person needs. These include carbohydrates, proteins, and fat. Other percent daily values – like those for sodium, potassium, vitamins, and minerals – stay the same no matter how many calories a person eats.

A quick reference to % Daily Value (%DV) is to keep in mind that under 5% is low and over 20% is high.

Nutrients List: Nutrients to Limit

Calories and Calories from Fat: Calories tell us how much energy we are getting from a serving of this food. Many people eat more calories than they need without getting the recommended intakes for a number of important nutrients. This is where understanding the food label comes into play. Another important part of the label is the number of calories that come from fat. It is important to look at this because it's good to limit fat intake. Calories in food can come from fat, protein, or carbohydrate.

Total Fat: The total fat is the number of grams of fat contained in one serving of the food. Fat is an important nutrient for growth and development, but you don't want to eat too much. The different kinds of fat, such as saturated, unsaturated, and trans fat, may be listed separately on the label.

Cholesterol and Sodium: These numbers tell you how much cholesterol and sodium (salt) are in a single serving of the food. They are included on the label because some people need to limit cholesterol or salt in their diets perhaps because they have high blood pressure, etc.

Total Carbohydrate: This number tells you how many carbohydrate grams are in one serving of food. This total is broken down into grams of sugar and grams of dietary fibre.

Protein: This number tells you how much protein you get from a single serving of the food. Your body needs protein to build and repair essential parts of the body, such as muscles, blood, and organs.

Nutrients List: Nutrients you want

Vitamins A and C: These list the amounts of vitamin A and vitamin C, two especially important vitamins, in a serving of the food. Each amount is given as a percent daily value. If a food provides 20% of the RDA for vitamin A, that one serving of food gives an adult one fifth of the vitamin A needed for the day.

Calcium and Iron: These list the percentages of calcium and iron, two especially important minerals that are in a serving of the food. Again, each amount is given as a percent daily value. If a food has 4% of iron, you're getting 4% of the iron you need for the whole day from that serving.

Eating strategies to help your child lose weight

Healthy Meals: It is your responsibility to make sure that your child is eating three well-balanced meals of average proportion each day. Choose fewer fatty foods and prepare meals that are baked, broiled or steamed, rather than fried. Do not forget your veggies; get your small serving of lean meat and your large serving of vegetables.

One Helping Only: One serving of the main course and dessert is sufficient. If you are still hungry, fill your plate up with more salad and other vegetables.

Desserts: Fresh fruit and yogurt served as a dessert is most healthy. Avoid high calorie desserts like ice cream or cake.

Grocery shopping: Choose low-calorie and lowfat meals, snacks and desserts. Avoid buying high calorie desserts or snacks, such as snack chips, regular soft drinks or regular ice cream.

Eat at the table: Make a mealtime routine of sitting down at the kitchen or dining room table. Even when it comes to snack time, it is best to eat these in the kitchen as well. And most important – no eating while watching TV!

No Fast Food: Make limits on how often you allow your children to eat fast food. These foods are high in calories and fat, and very low in nutrients.

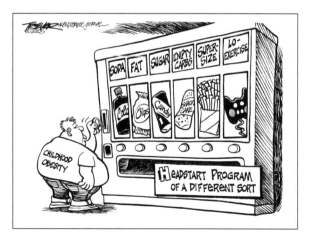

Proper nutrition and the ability to learn

Good nutrition and learning march hand-in-hand. Children who are balanced nutritionally are more likely to have the energy, stamina and self-esteem to enhance their ability to learn. Their minds are filled with thoughts of playing with their friends, joining clubs, participating in sports and (hopefully) getting good grades – children are not paying much attention to proper nutrition needed to accomplish all of this things. So where do you start?

We all know very well that breakfast is the most important meal of the day, yet almost half of adults skip breakfast. The statistics for children are just as alarming with almost identical trends as their breakfast-skipping parents. For many other children, breakfast is a trip to a convenience store or a vending machine for a soda pop and a high-fat, high-sugar snack. These are not ideal meal choices, nor does the price of having them come cheap. To help ensure that their child receives proper nutrition before heading out to school parents need to follow some simple nutrition rules.

Begin their day with a healthy breakfast. For school-aged children, a morning meal is especially important to prepare them to meet the challenges of learning. Many studies have shown that those who eat a morning meal tend to perform better in school, score higher on tests, have higher school attendance, less tardiness, better concentration and better muscle coordination. Children who eat breakfast also have fewer hunger-induced stomachaches and are less likely to be overweight or obese.

The importance of breakfast

Breakfast can be made fun by planning it out with your child. First decide who is going to prepare what and work with them to get it accomplished. One good example would be eggs, whole grain toast with nut butter, and a piece of fruit. Tofu or lean meat are good choices as well. Eating a breakfast consisting of protein and lower-starch foods will keep your child feeling more satisfied until lunch time. If your child doesn't like traditional breakfast foods, don't worry – breakfast can be any food they like.

Do not offer sugary breakfast options as they will leave your child hungry and tired throughout the morning. If your child is not hungry in the morning, start them out with something light like juice and whole-grain toast with peanut butter or almond butter and send them off with a nutritious mid-morning snack such as yogurt, cheese, an apple or a whole-grain bagel rather than sugary cookies or a pastry.

Some children believe that they will lose weight if they skip breakfast. Just the opposite is true. This trend in meal skipping often reflects in poorer eating habits later in the day such as overeating once they get home from school until they go to bed. Having too much unsatisfied hunger during the day can lead to moodiness, irritability, and an over-all inability to concentrate. Another downfall to skipping meals and letting yourself get very hungry before you eat is that you lose the ability to sense the feeling of fullness, and you don't stop eating when you are full. This can result in consuming more calories than if you had eaten an appropriate breakfast.

A study by Harvard University and Massachusetts General Hospital of children in Philadelphia and Baltimore showed that children who regularly ate breakfast had better standardized test scores, better behavior, and were less hyperactive than children who skipped breakfast. Another study at Oxford University in London compared low Glycemic Index (GI) breakfasts to high GI breakfasts which were consumed by 9-12 year old children. The children who ate the high GI breakfasts (sugary breakfasts) tended to eat more at lunch. It is the opinion of the researchers that low GI breakfasts could be an important factor for controlling obesity in children.

Lunchtime at school

While you cannot stop your child from the temptation of trading snacks or lunches with friends, you can send them to school with wholesome, nutritious food that satisfies them. Although many schools try to offer nutritious lunches, just as many still offer fast food, greasy pizzas, french fries, and other foods with low nutritional value.

Pack lunches that are easy to prepare and fun to eat. Involving your child in this process will increase the odds that they will resist trading their carrots for cookies. Some examples are sandwiches, raw veggies, crackers, string cheese, whole fruit and yogurt or pudding.

Good school lunches include hearty soups, salads, fruits, and sandwiches with whole grains, packed in insulated containers to stay hot or cold. Getting healthy nutrition at lunch time will help keep your child's mind sharp and ready to learn all afternoon.

After school snacks

Even with a great breakfast and healthy lunch, a light after-school snack is nice to refuel a child's body before play or study-time. Choose foods that supply necessary nutrients that can be missed in meal choices. Stock your refrigerator and pantry with ready-to-eat fruits and vegetables, whole-grain crackers, nuts, and even ingredient for a healthy version of a peanut butter and jelly sandwich (whole-grain bread, almond butter, and sugar-free jam) will satisfy picky kids. Your child will appreciate the availability of quick healthy snacks. Do not bring chips or candy in the house, as sugary and high Glycemic Index foods just make kids more hungry.

Life-long health through good nutrition

Studies show that overweight children tend to become overweight adults. Teach your children about healthy foods. Have them help you plan a meal which includes a healthy serving of protein, a vegetable or two, and a healthy fruit for dessert. For younger children, you can even keep a chart on the refrigerator to keep track of all the fruits and vegetables they eat and reward them with stickers or stamps when they choose healthy snacks. Snack time can be more fun if you try different recipes and snack ideas together with your kids.

Proper nutrition is crucial for social, emotional and psychological development. Teaching your children to how to have a healthy diet will have a bigger impact if you set the example. Eat right, exercise regularly, and make a healthy lifestyle a Fit Family affair.

Supplement recommendations
For those who WON'T eat breakfast

Whether it's the kids or yourself who won't eat breakfast, a health shake might be the right intermediate step. The *No Nonsense Diet*® with PGX® is a clinically proven, completely safe, natural, and highly effective way to achieve and maintain weight loss. Because of PGX®, a unique blend of soluble fibres, *No Nonsense Diet*® diminishes appetite, so you will eat less, without effort. Use *No Nonsense Diet*® shakes to:

- Reduce cravings – curb appetite
- Diet without hunger – stay full and satisfied for hours
- Balance and help regulate blood sugar
- Suitable for low-carb and reduced calorie diets – packed with nutrition
- Very low glycemic index/gluten free
- Delicious all natural sweeteners and flavours

What is PGX® and how does it help with weight?

PGX® is the acronym for PolyGlycopleX and is the key component of the *No Nonsense Diet*® Program. PGX® is a proprietary blend of soluble and indigestible fibres developed through several years of research at the University of Toronto. Clinical research has shown that PGX® fibre thickens and expands in your stomach and intestines, creating a sense of fullness that effectively controls appetite for several hours. After using PGX® for several days, most people will report that their appetite is lessened and their food cravings are greatly decreased.

In addition to its appetite-regulating properties, PGX® can also assist in balancing glucose and insulin levels. Insulin is an important hormone produced by the pancreas and it helps transport sugar from the blood stream into cells were it is burned for energy. Normally the body maintains a careful balance between glucose and insulin. However, most overweight individuals suffer from a condition known as insulin resistance, a condition in which insulin loses its effectiveness and high levels of insulin are produced by the pancreas. If unchecked, insulin resistance can lead to greater weight gain, food cravings, and an increased risk of developing diabetes along with a host of problems such as high blood pressure, elevated cholesterol levels and cardiovascular disease.

Why add whey protein?

Whey protein is another vital ingredient that assists with weight management. Like PGX®, whey protein helps provide a sense of fullness by increasing an appetite suppressing hormone known as CCK (Cholecystokinin). Increasing protein intake along with a low calorie diet and regular exercise has been shown to help promote both fat loss and healthy muscle growth.

In addition to macronutrients like whey and PGX®, the *No Nonsense Diet®* also incorporates specific nutrients that help maintain healthy glycemic levels, including:

Vitamin/Mineral	Action
Vitamin E	antioxidant
Vitamin C	antioxidant
Chromium	glucose tolerance factor
Zinc	supports chromium
Magnesium	supports chromium
Selenium	works synergistically with vitamin E

How to use the No Nonsense Diet® and meal replacement program:

The *No Nonsense Diet®* and meal replacement program is usually taken twice a day at breakfast and lunch along with a lower calorie, regular dinner. Healthy, low glycemic snacks should be taken three times a day: mid-morning, mid-afternoon, and mid-evening to help control cravings. Used as directed, the *No Nonsense Diet®* meal replacement works with your menu plan and regular exercise program for weight loss success.

As PGX® absorbs large amounts of water and expands in the intestine you must drink at least an additional 375–500 mL of water every time you use the meal replacement. Prescription medications should be taken at least 1 to 2 hours apart from any product containing PGX® fibre.

*"The art of medicine consists of amusing the patient
while nature cures the disease."*
Voltaire

CHAPTER 6

Detoxification

Do you ever feel sluggish? As if your body has to work extra hard just to function? As if stress were something you could measure by the pound? Every day the average North American is exposed to hundreds of different toxins, substances that actually create extra work for the body's detoxification systems. Toxins exist everywhere and can lead to serious health problems. They are in food and the environment, and they stay in our bodies. They can drain the body of energy and make you more susceptible to disease and infection. Toxins tend to concentrate in the liver and gastrointestinal tract, both places responsible for eliminating toxins from the body. Since everyone is exposed to toxins, everyone can use a detoxification treatment on a regular basis. People who are overweight are very often "holding" toxins in fatty deposits, which can make it even more difficult for the body to function and burn fat.

What is detoxification?

Detoxification is the process of deactivating and removing toxic substances from the body. A toxin is any substance that has a negative effect on cellular functions or structures in the body. Toxins can enter our body through our diet, from prescription medications, and environmental exposure. Toxins also exist in our bodies as a result of metabolic processes such as fat and cholesterol oxidation, and free radical formation. Because the liver, kidneys, lungs, skin, and intestines are the major organs of detoxification, toxic overload can be increased by poor digestion, colon sluggishness and dysfunction, reduced liver function, and by poor elimination through the kidneys, respiratory tract, and skin. Detoxification can also help remove any excess 'good' bio-chemicals, such as estrogen and testosterone.

The process of detoxification involves dietary and lifestyle changes to reduce the intake of toxins and improve elimination. It is very important to avoid chemicals, from food or other sources, refined food, sugar, caffeine, alcohol, and tobacco to help minimize the toxin load. Drinking plenty of water and increasing dietary fibre are important steps to support detoxification.

Why should I detox?

There are many reasons to detoxify or cleanse our bodies – mainly to do with health, vitality, and rejuvenation – to clear symptoms, treat disease, make a lifestyle change, and as a good start to a weight loss program. Detoxification can be helpful for weight loss, though it is not to be used primarily for weight loss alone. However, anyone eating 4,000 calories a day of a fatty, sweet, and poorly balanced diet who then begins to eat 2,000 to 2,500 calories of more wholesome foods will definitely experience detoxification, weight loss, and improved health.

Detoxifying is also important to rest overloaded organs and allow them to catch up on past work. An effective detox program can increase energy, reduce weight and eliminate subtle and mysterious chronic symptoms of non-optimum health.

When is the best time/season to detox?

Choosing a the right time to begin a detoxification program can be a challenge. It is important to incorporate nature's cycles with our own cycles. At certain times of the year you may notice regular periods of congestion, and may reduce or prevent these by beginning a detoxification program. A period of congestion may include the start of a cold, at which time exercising, sweating, saunas or steam, drinking lots of fluids, taking vitamin C, and a good night's sleep, can begin the detoxification process.

What changes can I expect?

The effects of a detoxification diet vary from person to person. Making even small changes to your current diet may produce some responses, but more dramatic dietary alterations will produce a much more profound detoxification. Remarkable things can happen when you improve the quality of food you eat and take better care of your body and more specifically, your organs. At this time, more rest and sleep is often needed. It is also imperative to avoid stimulants of any kind (alcohol, caffeine, drugs) which will abort and defeat the regenerative process. Remember the body isn't getting weaker. It's simply using its energies in more important internal work, rather than external work involving muscle movements. Be patient. You will soon feel more energy than before.

When you stop drinking coffee or chocolate you may experience headaches and a sense of fatigue. Your body begins discarding toxins such as caffeine and theobromine by removing them from the tissues and transporting them through the bloodstream. However, before toxins are eliminated, they register as a headache. These symptoms are part of a healing process that is constructive even if unpleasant. Ensuring that your body receives sufficient nutrition (perhaps supplementing with *No Nonsense Diet*® shakes for example) can ease any unpleasant side effects of detoxification.

Such symptoms become milder and pass more quickly, as detoxification progresses, as long as you get enough rest and sleep. The body becomes healthier by eliminating waste and toxins. These stored toxins eventually could cause or contribute to illness and disease.

Detoxification you can do at home

I have touched on ways to detoxify throughout this section; the remainder is a discussion of general and specific diet plans, other activities, and supplements, including vitamins, minerals, amino acids, and herbs, to support this healing process.

There are many levels to this part of the program. The first is to eat a non-toxic diet. If you do this regularly, you will have less need for cleansing. If you have not been eating this way, detoxify first and then make permanent changes.

Hydrotherapy

The benefits of "water healing," or hydrotherapy have been recognized for thousands of years. Water healing is one of the oldest, least expensive and safest methods for treating many common ailments, including aiding the detoxification process.

Contrast showers

The contrast between hot and cold water increases the circulation in the body, promotes detoxification, and strengthens the immune system. This stimulation helps bring nutrients, oxygen and immune cells to damaged tissues and flushes out metabolic waste and toxic substances. Contrast showers also strengthen the immune system by increasing the number of white blood cells.

How to do a contrast shower

Begin the shower three minutes of hot water followed by less than one minute of cold water. Repeat this cycle at least once and always finish with cold water (e.g. 3 minutes hot – 1 minute cold – 3 minutes hot – 1 minute cold). Ending your shower with cold water helps to return blood flow to your internal organs.

Castor Oil Pack

Castor Oil has traditionally been known as a strong laxative when taken internally. A more gentle use of it is in the form of an external application of a pack placed over the abdomen with heat. The oil is absorbed into the lymphatic circulation to provide a soothing, cleansing, and nutritive treatment, which stimulates immune function and tonifies internal organs.

Extremely sensitive patients, such as those with multiple chemical sensitivities, may experience an increase in their symptoms. I would not recommend using castor oil packs in pregnancy or during menstruation as it may create additional bleeding. Contact your naturopathic doctor for your specific situation.

Materials:

- castor oil
- 2 sheets of plastic (garbage bags OK)
- 36" x 18" white cotton flannel or wool flannel
- hot water bottle or heating pad
- old sheet, wool blanket, pillows
- baking soda

Procedure:

1. Fold flannel into 2-3" thickness to fit over your entire abdomen.
2. Soak flannel with the castor oil. Fold flannel in half and strip excess oil from pack. Unfold. The first few times you use it, it will seem there is too much oil present. However, be patient and usually after several applications, the flannel will have just the right amount of castor oil.
3. Apply to abdomen and put an opened plastic bag or piece of plastic wrap on top of the flannel (to avoid staining). Castor oil stains and you will not be likely to get it out, so be cautious.
4. Then wrap abdomen with an old towel so it overlaps at front.
5. Tie this comfortably tight by using 2 ace bandages, one around the ribs and the other around the waist, to keep the pack close to the body.
6. Apply heating pad over this to maintain heat.
7. Wrap up in a robe/gown and read or relax for 45 minutes to an hour. This is an excellent time to practice visualization, meditation or relaxation breathing.
8. After finishing, you can leave the oil on the skin to be absorbed or, to remove the oil, wash with a solution of 2 tablespoons of baking soda to 1 quart water.

Store the pack in a large zip-lock bag (which you may keep in the fridge). Reuse the pack many times, adding more oil as needed to keep the pack saturated. Replace the pack after it begins to change colour (usually several months).

Use the pack as often as possible; patients who use the pack daily will receive the most beneficial effects.

Herbs to support detoxification

For the colon, the following herbs are generally indicated during a cleanse:

Psyllium is well known for its gentle effect on the intestines and its capacity to form a soft-bulky stool that stimulates bowel movement.

Chlorella and Spirulina are traditional herbal sources of chlorophyll, which is absorbed into the blood and binds to circulating toxic molecules and heavy metals, for urine elimination. They also increase bowel fibre which binds to conjugated toxins.

Cascara sagrada is a mild stimulation laxative, which facilitates bile elimination through increased bowel movements.

Slippery Elm has a demulcent or soothing effect on the intestinal tract.

Ginger Root provides an antispasmodic action and reduces the tendency for gas or bloating. It stimulates production of bile and acts as a potent anti-inflammatory agent to protect the liver from injury.

Liver cleansing herbs generally include:

Milk Thistle is a potent liver health enhancer, stimulating production of glutathione, protecting and enhancing liver health. It also stimulates the liver to regenerate injured cells, returning lost performance capacity.

Globe Artichoke stimulates the production of bile to enhance bile elimination of conjugated-toxins and, as a natural diuretic, it increases urine elimination.

Dandelion Root increases the production of bile and increases its flow to the intestines and also acts as a mild diuretic.

Burdock Root is thought to stimulate pancreatic function, enhancing digestion and reducing food putrefaction toxins. It is also used to facilitate liver lymphatic drainage which can improve liver function.

Red Clover stimulates liver detoxification. It is known as a treatment for eczema and psoriasis.

As with pharmaceutical medications, herbs and supplements should be used with caution, especially during pregnancy. If you have an adverse reaction to an herb or supplement, stop using it immediately and report your condition to your local pharmacist and naturopathic doctor. Always consult your health-care practitioner for proper dosage, and any contraindications if you are taking prescription medications, and before altering your treatment or beginning a detoxification program.

The Fit Family Program and Detoxification

By following the Fit Family Program, you are well on your way to a body that is continually detoxifying itself and not storing loads of toxins.

- Encourage your family to eat foods that resemble their natural state and are not processed or refined.

- Eliminate all the foods that are having a negative impact on your health – sugar, caffeine, alcohol, preservatives, red meat, canned foods, saturated fats, and tobacco.

- Choose your fluids more wisely. Simply increasing liquids and decreasing fats will shift the balance strongly toward improved elimination and less toxin buildup.

- Start out your day with hot water with lemon to promote liver detoxification rather than your typical morning coffee.

- Increase your water intake to help flush toxins out of your body.

- Especially during your detoxification program, choose organic foods which are free of pesticides.

- Cook in iron, stainless steel, glass, or porcelain.

- Drink green tea, a dietary source of catechin, and other herbal teas.

- Eat a well-balanced diet rich in fresh fruits and vegetables.

- Eat artichokes, which help detox the liver.

· Eat foods in the Brassica family (cabbage, cauliflower, brussel sprouts).

· Increase intake of berries.

· Most importantly, keep a food diary to detect individual patterns of sensitivity to foods.

Maintaining the Fit Family program while adding detoxifying supplements can have an additive effect on your detoxification process.

Supplement recommendations

I have found the following products to be particularly effective, and gentle. They can be used to simplify the detoxification process.

PureBody™ Detox Kit (Liver Cleanse & Colon Cleanse)

The PureBody Detoxification System is an herb-based system, designed to enhance detoxification by:

· strengthening your liver's own health and load capacity

· facilitating improved elimination.

You can use the PureBody Detoxification System 2-3 times a year to enhance health, vitality, improve digestion and energy levels. PureBody is not a fasting program, but a gentle colon and liver cleanse.

Colon Cleanse

Three natural fibres in Colon Cleanse improve bowel movement patterns required for toxin-loaded bile elimination: Psyllium, well known for its gentle effect on the intestines and its capacity to form a soft-bulky stool that stimulates bowel movement; Chlorella and Spirulina, traditional herbal sources of chlorophyll, which is absorbed into the blood and binds to circulating toxic molecules and heavy metals, for urine elimination. They also increase bowel fibre which binds to conjugated toxins.

Liver Cleanse

This aspect of the PureBody™ program contains: Milk Thistle, a potent liver health enhancer, which also stimulates the liver to regenerate injured cells, regaining performance capacity; Globe Artichoke, stimulates production of bile to enhance bile elimination of conjugated-toxins and, as a natural diuretic, it increases urine flow; Dandelion Root increases production of bile and its flow to the intestines and acts as a mild diuretic; Burdock Root is thought to stimulate pancreatic function, enhancing digestion and reducing food putrefaction toxins. It is also used to facilitate liver lymphatic drainage which can improve liver function; Red Clover stimulates liver detoxification. It is known as a treatment for eczema and psoriasis; Cascara sagrada is a mild stimulation laxative, which facilitates bile elimination through increased bowel movements; Slippery Elm has a demulcent or soothing effect on the intestinal tract; Ginger Root provides an antispasmodic action and reduces the tendency for gas or bloating effects, also acts as a potent anti-inflammatory agent to protect the liver from injury.

Webber naturals™ Acidophilus & Bifidus (Non-Dairy)

This probiotic supplement is a combination of friendly lactic acid bacteria that colonize the intestinal tract for better digestive health. Acidophilus produces lactic acid that keeps a proper pH balance in the small intestine, slowing the growth of yeast. Bifidus helps maintain health of the large intestine in both children and adults, promoting regular bowel movements, protecting from yeast and bacteria such as E.coli, Clostridium and Shigella.

"In the midst of movement and chaos,
keep stillness inside of you."
Deepak Chopra

CHAPTER 7

Stress management

Stressed out? Fed up? You're not alone. Stress is a clear message to change something in our lives for the better. Stress has become an accepted part of life for many people, and a common factor in many illnesses. Of deaths that occur prematurely, a large portion of them are stress-related, with coronary heart disease leading the pack. We are literally working ourselves to death – is it worth it?

Understanding how stress relates to health is an important part of understanding how to manage it. We can't always control what stressful events might occur in our lives, but we can take actions to minimize the impact on our health.

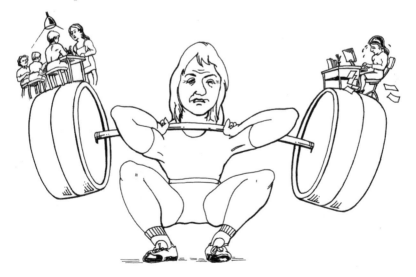

What is stress?

Stress is your body's reaction to events in your life. There exist both 'good' stress and 'bad' stress. A rush of adrenaline when we are experiencing good stress can be exhilarating and fulfilling, yet too much all at once can be overwhelming. How stress affects you depends on how well-equipped you are to respond in any given situation. World-recognized stress researcher, Hans Seyle, MD, remarked that, "The same stress event which makes one person sick can be an invigorating experience for another."

Seconds after a stressful event or an acutely dangerous moment, your adrenal glands release hormones (epinephrine and norepinephrine) into your bloodstream to prepare your body to deal with this stress. These hormones will suppress normal body functions such as digestion, while enhancing your heart rate and increasing sweating to start the FIGHT or FLIGHT response. Almost immediately your adrenal glands release extra cortisol into circulation. Once the stressful event has passed, hormone levels and body functions return to a normal, balanced state.

Your body's response to stress is essential to survival. Every day you learn to adapt to an ever-changing environment. However, your body's stress response can become a problem when it is kicking into action on a daily basis, or even multiple times during the day. This type of chronic stress can lead to many health problems because you are constantly depleting your body's reserves. You may begin to feel "stressed out" and like "you have only one nerve left...". You are jeopardizing your health if you allow stress to dominate your daily life.

What triggers stress?

Stress can be triggered by many things, including some you might not expect!

Emotional Stress	Anger	Anxiety
Death of spouse	Divorce	Marriage
Losing a job	Retirement	Pregnancy
Financial Problems	Vacations	Physical Stress
Accidents	Burns	Surgery
Over-exercising	Poor sleep	Obesity
Environmental Stress	Pesticides	Allergies
Noise	Pollution	Metabolic Stress
Nutrient deficiencies due to diet or prescription medications	Oxidative stress – free radical formation (i.e. smoking)	Poor diet (high sugar, high fat)

Early Warning Signs that Stress May Be Affecting Your Health

Fatigue	Irritability	Depression
Disturbed Sleep	Negative Attitude	Over-Eating
Alcohol Consumption	Dependence on alcohol or cigarettes to unwind	Poor Immune System (frequent colds/coughs)

Stress and your immune system

A healthy immune system regulates our body's ability to heal and protects it against infections and diseases. When stress compromises immune function, it can result in colds, flu, fatigue, cardiovascular disorders and premature aging. Stress increases heart rate, blood pressure, glucose levels, adrenaline, cortisol, free radicals and oxidative damage. This initiates the fight or flight response, places undue strain upon the heart, and can also increase the feelings of anxiety and depression. Bouts of acute stress in any form can cause a temporary decrease in functioning of the immune system, while chronic stress will result in a continued decline in function over time.

Digestive disturbances and stress

Stress has a significant impact on the digestive system. Not only can stressful events disrupt the digestive process, but reducing stress can provide relief of some digestion-related disorders such as gastric acid secretion, chronic diarrhea, irritable bowel syndrome, and peptic ulcers. When we experience stress our nutritional needs change to can help the body "cope" by providing enough of certain nutrients that are in greater demand or are more difficult to acquire when we perceive stress. Relaxation techniques, nutritional supplementation are often used to provide relief.

Stress busters

During times of increased or prolonged stress, nutritional and botanical therapies can help us cope:

- B vitamins, magnesium, zinc, vitamin C, Siberian ginseng (Eleutherococcus senticosis) and Panax ginseng support adrenal function.

- Antioxidants fight and neutralize free radicals, which are molecules that damage cells and cause heart disease, cancer and premature aging.

- Omega-3 fatty acids (a polyunsaturated fat) have anti-inflammatory, cardiovascular-enhancing and immune-regulating properties. These are helpful in preventing and controlling high cholesterol, hypertension, heart disease, stroke, cancer, diabetes, depression, inflammatory and auto-immune disorders.

- Folate prevents age-related cognitive decline, damage to blood vessels and brain cells by lowering homocysteine levels. It also ensures DNA integrity (important as we age and when pregnant) and promotes healthy red blood cells.

Controlling your weight, in a healthy way, can greatly reduce emotional and physical stresses. The physical stress on your body from carrying too much weight can be relieved and higher self esteem definitely improves your reaction to stressful situations. The key is to give your body good nutrition consistently and remove factors and lifestyle elements that push you into unhealthy habits.

Fit Family Plan dietary recommendations

Maintain a diet of mostly whole (unprocessed) foods.

Avoid Caffeine. Caffeine causes a fight-or- flight response in your body and uses up your reserves of the B vitamins, which are important in coping with stress. Caffeine (coffee, tea, cola, chocolate) also causes nervousness and inhibits sleep if too much is ingested.

Avoid alcohol. Alcohol also depletes your body's B vitamins, and can disrupt sleep and impair your judgment or clarity of thought.

Avoid sugar. It provides no essential nutrients and can cause an immediate energy high, followed by a prolonged low.

Eat foods rich in antioxidants (vitamins A, C, E and lycopene), omega-3 fatty acids, and folate. Excellent food sources for these nutrients are:

- Antioxidants – pumpkin, sweet potatoes, carrots, kale, grapefruit (red and pink), blueberries, strawberries, watermelon, cantaloupe, oranges, peppers (red and green), tomatoes, broccoli, sunflower seeds, almonds and olive oil.

- Omega-3 Fatty Acids – fish oils, ground flax seeds, walnuts, soybeans and pumpkin seeds.

- Folate – dark green leafy vegetables (turnip greens, mustard greens, spinach, romaine lettuce, collard greens, etc.), beans, legumes, asparagus, Brussels sprouts, and beets

Sleep

Try to go to bed at the same time every day and get up at the same time every day. Every hour of sleep before 12:00 midnight is worth 2 hours after midnight. A good night's sleep will also improve your memory and help to balance your hormones.

Relaxation techniques

Deep Breathing – Lay flat on your back with your head lower than your body. With your left hand on your upper chest and your right hand on your stomach, inhale deeply through your nose and push outward with your stomach. Your right hand should feel your abdomen rise. Try to keep the left hand still while inhaling. Breathe in with your stomach muscles, not with your chest. Purse your lips and exhale slowly, pushing the abdomen in and up toward the ribs, feeling your right hand move as you do so. Try to exhale slowly for as long as you can, before inhaling again. Now that you have mastered this breathing technique, you can do this breathing at other times throughout the day. Aim to do 100 of these breaths every day.

Hydrotherapy – Relaxing in a hot bath relieves sore muscles and joints, reduces stress and tension, and promotes a good night's sleep. Add some Epsom salts to the bath, essential oils of your choice, soothing music, and soft lighting (candles are nice) to create a spa atmosphere in the comfort and privacy of your own home.

Music – Listening to your favourite music is a great method of reducing stress and relieving anxiety. Pay attention to how you feel when you hear a particular song or genre of music, and keep listening to the ones that produce a relaxing effect and help to lower your blood pressure.

Exercise

A circulation-enhancer, physical activity is essential for providing a sense of well-being and stress reduction. A regular exercise schedule which includes both cardio and strength training strengthens your immune system, cardiovascular system, heart, muscles, and bones. Exercise also stimulates the release of endorphins, improves mental focus and concentration, lowers cholesterol, blood pressure, cortisol, and other stress hormones. Daily exercise is essential. Three 10-minute workout sessions during the day are just as effective as one 30-minute workout, and a lot easier to fit into a busy schedule.

Yoga and Stretching – The slow movements and controlled postures of yoga improves muscle strength, flexibility, range of motion, balance, breathing, blood circulation and promotes mental focus, clarity and calmness. Stretching also reduces mental and physical stress, tension and anxiety, promotes good sleep, lowers blood pressure and slows down your heart rate.

Time management

When it's not possible to add extra hours to the day, it helps to spend time and energy on what's most important. It is much easier to focus our energies on concentrating on one thing at a time, so minimizing distractions and focusing on the task at hand can help us accomplish our goals more effectively. Organization and time management can minimize stress and maximize efficiency. Taking breaks during the day to stretch and change focus makes work hours more productive.

Play

Do something FUN everyday. There is truth to the saying that laughter is the best medicine. Laughter is essential for stress management and a healthy heart. Laughing reduces stress hormones like adrenaline (epinephrine) and cortisol. It also benefits your immune system by increasing the number and activity of Natural Killer T-cells. Working hard is commendable, but we also need to play.

Attitude

Remaining calm, cool and collected when addressing difficult situations is key to changing our experience of stress. Optimism can counteract the negative impact stress, tension and anxiety have on your immune system and well-being. Having a positive attitude, finding the good in life and looking at the bright side of things enhances your ability to effectively manage stress.

Supplement recommendations

If planning and making healthy meals is just another source of stress for you, be sure you supplement with the following nutrients to balance your diet if you eat out, resort to fast foods or skip meals from time to time:

Antioxidant Supplements

Some of the best sources of healthy antioxidants are:

AllGreens®: A powder or capsule form of nutrient dense plant foods.

Alpha-lipoic Acid: An essential enzyme involved in energy production, and an antioxidant that helps convert food into energy. It is both fat and water soluble, allowing it to quench free radicals both inside and outside the cell. It may help control blood sugar levels and have therapeutic application in managing diabetes.

Coenzyme Q10 (CoQ10): Low levels of CoQ10 have been associated with compromised immune function, gum disease and heart failure. CoQ10 100mg is a high potency antioxidant and a key nutrient to slow aging. May also be found in combination formulas with natural source Vitamin E.

Lutein and Zeaxanthin: These two carotenoids are particularly good at protecting the eyes, the arteries and the lungs from damaging free radicals. Dark green leafy vegetables like spinach and kale, are rich in lutein. Webber naturals™ FloraGlo® Lutein is made from marigold flowers with a concentration of lutein that is 20 times higher than spinach.

Vitamin E: A fat-soluble vitamin and a powerful antioxidant, protecting cell membranes from pollution, toxins and free radicals. Vitamin E is the major antioxidant in lipid (fatty) body tissues and the primary defense against lipid peroxidation, particularly in the brain and central nervous system. Natural source vitamin E, designated by the prefix d, (d-alpha-tocopherol) is almost twice as bioavailable as synthetic vitamin E, designated by the prefix dl (dl-alpha-tocopherol).

Vitamin C: the water soluble antioxidant most often used to support immunity. Although most people consume considerable amounts of dietary vitamin C, it cannot be stored by the body so supplementation offers good "insurance".

Other stress busting nutrients

B Vitamins: A good balance of the many B vitamins is essential for nerve health, stress control and a good night's sleep. Don't take B vitamins before bed however as they also contribute to energy production.

B 5 – Also known as Pantothenic acid, B 5 is converted in the body to coenzyme A, which is necessary for the metabolisms of fats, carbohydrates and proteins, and the synthesis of cholesteral, bile and steroids. Coenzyme A can detoxify harmful substances found in herbicides, insecticides, and drugs. D-pantothenic acid is considered an anti-stress vitamin because it is vital for the adrenal gland to function properly.

B 12, B 6 – Vitamin B12 (Cyanocobalamin) works with folic acid and vitamin B6 to control homocysteine levels. Research shows that high levels of homocysteine may dramatically increase the risk of heart disease and osteoporosis. Vitamin B12 is also important for nervous system function, memory and learning; for the synthesis of red blood cells and for producing the genetic materials, DNA and RNA. Vitamin B6 is often called "the woman's vitamin" as it is helpful for reducing PMS symptoms and may help relieve or prevent moodswings associated with the use of oral contraceptives.

Calcium and Magnesium are, of course, essential to healthy bones but they also help relax the muscles and improve sleep.

Stress relieving herbs

Standardized green tea extract contains highly purified polyphenols – plant chemicals that act as natural antioxidants and antimicrobial agents. The antioxidants help prevent free radical damage to cells, while cholesterol-lowering green tea polyphenols have been shown to reduce plaque buildup in the arteries and have a beneficial effect on high blood pressure. New studies show that green tea extract can help with weight loss as it speeds up metabolism.

Rhodiola is a new and effective herbal extract that works as an adaptogen to help manage stress. Rhodiola has six groups of chemical compounds that appear to work by inhibiting the breakdown of seratonin, dopamine and norepinephrine, thereby facilitating the transport and levels of these compounds in the brain. The effects help memory, learning, attention, and sleep, while reducing fatigue and stress.

St. John's Wort: Studies show that people taking St. John's Wort experience natural mood elevation and reduced feelings of sadness or hopelessness and often experience a better sleep pattern.

"Nature, time and patience are three great physicians."
H.G. Bohn

CHAPTER 8

Nutritional supplementation

Throughout this book I have made supplement recommendations to help with diet, stress and overall health. But I'm often asked, "Why do I need supplements?" So let's answer that question.

All human beings need adequate micronutrients (vitamins, minerals, enzymes and trace elements) for good health. Ideally, we would obtain all the necessary micronutrients from a well balanced diet. However, as we outlined in the first chapter, the nutritional quality of the food in our world has been steadily declining, particularly in the last century. In the past, people ate foods that were whole, fresh, in-season and grown locally in nutrient-dense soil. Now, most foods are refined, preserved and grown in nutrient-depleted soils, making it difficult for us to get all the nutrients we need solely from food, no matter how "nutritious" our diet may seem.

Many genetic, environmental and lifestyle factors also contribute to INCREASED nutrient requirements. Just as there is genetic variability in hair or eye colour, there is genetic variability in our requirements for, and abilities to absorb and use, certain nutrients. Some of us need more of certain vitamins or minerals in order to maintain optimal health. It is interesting to note that women who take supplements tend to weigh less than other women (Lin et al., 2004).

Another factor that affects our nutrient levels and requirements is pollution. Pollutants, pesticides and toxins are an unfortunate reality and the body's ability to protect itself from these substances is largely dependent on our nutritional status. Pollutants can interfere with specific vitamins, such as B6 and others, leading to deficiencies. Other factors including stress, activity levels, medications and illnesses can elevate an individual's requirements for certain vitamins and minerals.

RDI means "recommended daily intake" and RDA means "recommended daily allowance". These terms relate to the amount of a nutrient that is required to avoid developing a deficiency disease, such as scurvy (vitamin C deficiency) or rickets (vitamin D and calcium deficiency). This doesn't mean that the RDI is the optimum amount of any nutrient for an active healthy life.

Why supplement?

- To balance nutrient levels in the face of the declining nutrient content and increased refinement of our foods.

- To overcome increased nutrient demands placed on our bodies by disease, pregnancy, high stress or high activity levels.

- To counteract the negative effects of pollution and environmental toxins.

- To correct nutritional deficiencies caused by poor diet or prescription medications.

- To achieve optimum health and utilize the health-promoting effects of specific nutrients.

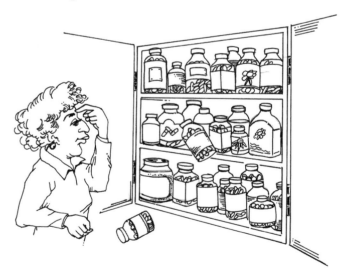

Nutritional supplements for the whole family

Vitamin C

What: Vitamin C is a powerful antioxidant and an important factor in immune system support and cardiovascular health. Antioxidants help to prevent or reduce damage to cells caused by free radicals.

Why: As well as being an antioxidant, vitamin C is necessary for maintaining all collagen structures. It also promotes wound healing, strong bones and teeth, and healthy gums. During times of stress, the body's need for vitamin C increases. Vitamin C acts as a powerful detoxifier, helping to cleanse the body of cigarette smoke and other damaging pollutants.

Since the body does not store vitamin C efficiently, it is important to be replaced daily. Choose Sunkist® Vitamin C to meet your vitamin C requirements and enhance your health.

Food sources: citrus fruits and juices, as well as in broccoli, red peppers, strawberries, tomatoes and potatoes.

A good multivitamin and multimineral formula

What: Multivitamin pills provide a full range of nutrients including vitamins, minerals, and trace elements that are important for maintaining health and replenishing nutrients that have been lost due to physical stress, poor diets and/or metabolic inefficiencies.

Why: Experts agree that taking a multivitamin is an excellent tool in the quest for good nutrition and better health. Unfortunately we are not getting enough of our vitamins and minerals from our diets. The processing, storing, or even cooking of foods can reduce the vitamin content. Foods can also be adversely affected by chemical fertilizers, pesticides, and poor soil conditions. In our bodies, nutrients are also negatively affected by heavy smoking, alcohol consumption, and numerous health conditions including chronic diseases and obesity.

Even if you follow Canada's Food Guide to Healthy Eating religiously, you still might need a multivitamin. Some vitamins have been shown to reduce the risks of cancer, heart disease and certain age-related illnesses, and it's not always easy to meet the recommended daily allowance (RDA) of some nutrients with food alone. Also, over time our bodies become less effective at absorbing some nutrients.

Essential Fatty Acids

What: Specific types of dietary fat that contribute to good health and are required in particular balance for optimum function.

Why: Omega-3 fatty acids are essential for a healthy cardiovascular system. Research suggests that increasing your consumption of omega-3 can reduce triglyceride levels and total cholesterol.

Essential fatty acids in general are extremely important in metabolism regulation, brain development and function, blood circulation, hemoglobin production and immune function. Along with lowering cholesterol and blood pressure, they also contribute to healthy skin, hair and nails, and help relieve some symptoms of PMS, especially breast tenderness and uterine cramping.

Essential fatty acids also have anti-inflammatory properties which researchers have found to benefit patients with rheumatoid arthritis. The same anti-inflammatory effect on the digestive tract has been credited with reducing symptoms and flare-ups of Crohn's disease and ulcerative colitis.

The typical North American diet is low in omega-3s. Experts believe that, for better health, we need to consume more of them. (See more about EFAs in Chapter 3.)

Food sources: Oily fish, such as salmon, trout, sardines, mackerel and herring, flaxseed oil, canola oil, walnuts and soybeans.

Acidophilus and Bifidus

What: These are "friendly" bacteria that live in the human intestinal tract.

Why: There are hundreds of bacteria that live in the digestive tract, the most beneficial being Lactobacillus acidophilus and L.bifidus. Acidophilus produces lactic acid which keeps a proper pH balance in the small intestine and slows the growth of yeast. Bifidus helps maintain the health and functioning of the large intestine in both children and adults, promoting regular bowel movements. Experts agree that consuming acidophilus and bifidus supplements aid in controlling vaginal yeast infections, as well as treating the symptoms of irritable bowel syndrome.

Food sources: fermented milk products, such as yogurt – or in nutritional supplements with varying strengths.

Supplement recommendations
Bone and Joint Health
Calcium is the most abundant mineral in the body, essential for building strong bones and teeth. The diets of most Canadian adults, however, are calcium poor and osteoporosis is extremely common among women, and men, as they age.

To prevent this bone-thinning disease requires a lifetime of adequate calcium intake from our diets as well as from supplements. Our body only builds bone up to the age of 35, however with a calcium-rich diet and supplements, we can help to maintain our bone density and decrease the risk of bone fractures.

When taking a calcium supplement, it is best to take it in combination with vitamin D and magnesium as these two nutrients work together with calcium to promote healthy bones.

Dairy products, such as milk, yogurt and cheese, are excellent sources of calcium. If you are lactose-intolerant, tofu, beans, broccoli, and dark green leafy vegetables, are good nondairy choices.

Glucosamine and Chondroitin sulfates are key building blocks of cartilage in the joints. The body naturally manufactures glucosamine and chondroitin, however this manufacturing decreases as we age. Significant scientific research and evidence exists to support the use of glucosamine and chondroitin to reduce symptoms of osteoarthritis and to slow the progression of the disease. In some patients it eases the pain and inflammation caused by osteoarthritis, increases the range of motion and helps to repair joints in the knees, hips, spine and hands.

Recent research by the National Institute of Health in their Glucosamine/chondroitin Arthritis Intervention Trial (GAIT) has compared the effects of glucosamine, chondroitin, the combination of the two as well as a COX-2 inhibitor to relieve arthritis symptoms. Results suggest that the combination of glucosamine and chondroitin were found to be more effective than Celebrex® in treating moderate to severe knee pain.

Celadrin™ is a medically and clinically proven compound of "esterified fatty acid carbons" (EFACs). It helps repair, restore, protect and lubricate cell membranes, providing fast relief for painful joints, muscles and tissues.

Damage to cells is at the root of all degenerative conditions. Celadrin™ enhances the function and integrity of cells by providing an ideal blend of lipids (fats) to repair and strengthen cell tissues and improve elasticity. Using Celadrin™ as a dietary supplement helps cell membranes remain efficient, fluid, permeable and "youthful". In a double blind clinical trial, Celadrin™ showed significant benefit beyond the arthritis medication the subjects were taking – with cumulative improvement throughout the study. Celadrin™ may be used safely with prescription medications and with other joint support supplements such as glucosamine and chondroitin.

Not all Celadrin™ products are equal. I suggest using one with a high concentration of EFACs, such as webber naturals™ 350 mg Celadrin™ softgel capsules, as they deliver as much or more than most 500 mg tablets.

*"Those who do not find time for exercise
will have to find time for illness"*
Earl of Derby

CHAPTER 9

Fitness for life

It may not be your favourite truth, but an essential part of any weight loss or weight management program is regular fitness. Let's look at the benefits of exercise and just how much exercise is enough.

Principle #1: Aerobic conditioning

Aerobic means "living, active, or occurring only in the presence of oxygen". It relates to exercises that increase respiration and heart rate, as compared to weight or strength training. Walking and running are the most common and popular ways to get the benefits of aerobic activity.

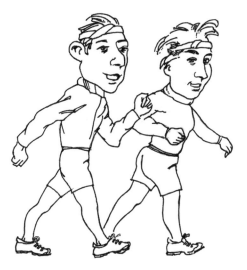

Walking tips

You may not think you need to be told how to walk, but try these tips to make your walking more "productive" as part of your fitness routine:

- Bend your elbows. Your arms will swing faster which will help your legs move faster too.
- Keep your stride short. Don't take long strides that feel awkward.
- Think heel-to-toe. Push-off with your heel. Toes should leave the ground last.
- Keep your abs pulled in and tight.
- Include interval training walks, that is periods of very brisk walking followed by slower walking for recovery.

Running tips

- If you are new to running you should start by walking for 30 minutes at least 3 days a week, about 3 months, before you make the move to running.
- Do not bounce or overstride. Don't let your foot get ahead of your knee. Run from the hips down, with the upper body straight up and used only for balance.
- Breathe in through your nose and out through pursed lips.
- Choose shoes appropriate for running and that fit well, to prevent discomfort or blisters.
- When running in colder weather be sure to wear a hat. A large amount of heat can be lost through your head.
- Replace your running shoes at least every 400-500 miles.

Principle #2: Strength training

Include some type of strength training in your weekly exercise regimen no matter what your fitness goals are. Resistance training provides many health benefits. Don't take the all or nothing approach. It's better to do a little training than none at all. So, even if you can only fit one strength training routine in a week, you'll still benefit from it.

If you're a woman, don't be afraid of strength training. You won't bulk up (unless you are really trying to) and resistance training is easy to start. With professional guidance and direction, you can quickly learn how to train properly.

Some strength training tips:

· Be sure you are training with the proper resistance size. Choose a size that fatigues you after 10-12 reps.

· Focus on correct form. If you are unable to use proper, safe form when performing an exercise then you probably are using weights that are too heavy. Choose a size that allows you to train with correct form.

· Concentrate on the muscle(s) you are working during a specific exercise and don't use other muscle groups to assist with the exercise.

· How long you rest between sets is important. For building muscles and getting bulkier the rest time should be longer. For more muscle endurance and leaner, sculpted muscles the rest time should be shorter.

· The frequency of your strength training depends on whether your goals are to get bigger and stronger (less often) or whether you want to get leaner and more defined muscles (more often).

Principle #3: Flexibility

Stretching and flexibility are very important aspects of good physical fitness, so don't overlook them. Ideally, you should stretch before each workout (both cardio and resistance exercises) and after. If you can't do both, make the after stretching a priority.

When stretching before a workout, it's best to stretch after you've warmed-up for about 5 minutes (your muscles will be looser).

Fit Family tips to increase your family's activity level

· Walk or ride your bikes instead of driving short distances.

· Walk with a friend or walk the family dog each afternoon.

· Use stairs instead of escalators or elevators.

· Park your car at the back of the parking lot and walk to the entrance of the mall or grocery store.

· Encourage regular exercise for 20-30 minutes 4-5 times each week. This can include walking, jogging, swimming, bike riding, rollerblading, riding a skateboard, etc.

· Try a new sport, such as basketball, volleyball, tennis, soccer, etc.

· Go for regular family walks or bike rides in your neighborhood or local park.

More exercise & workout tips

· Stair climbing is a low-impact alternative to running.

· Choose exercises that you enjoy doing. You'll be more inclined to stick with a fitness regimen when it includes things you like to do.

· Change your fitness routine every 4-6 weeks to prevent a work-out plateau.

· Strive to include total body workouts. These include: cardiovascular exercises, strength training (both upper and lower body), core training and stretching/flexibility.

Conclusion

Since the beginning of time, humans have had interesting and varied relationships with food. Can't live without it, but can't always live well with the kinds of food we choose to eat. In this book I have tried to give you some facts, some helpful tips and recommendations, and some guidance for a long, healthy life based on an intelligent and responsible relationship with food and fitness.

There is no magic bullet for a perfect body and little likelihood of consuming 100% proper nutrition every day, but there are basic principles you can follow, and there are new scientifically validated nutritional products that can definitely make it easier for you to make the changes needed for a slimmer, healthier YOU.

I encourage you to use this information to achieve your weight loss goals, to improve the health of your family, and to reduce the impact of stress on your daily life, so you can go beyond dieting and start living!

Dr. Joyce Tellier Johnson, ND

Bibliography

The preceding information has been extracted from, *Effects of conjugated linoleic acid in humans from Scandinavian Clinical Research AS*, Kjeller, Norway, as well as Review of the Scientific and Clinical Data on the Health Benefits of CLA by Delbert R. Dorscheid, MD, Ph.D.

American Diabetes Association. Consensus Development Conference on Insulin Resistance. November 5-6, 1997. Diabetes Care 1998;21:310-4.

Colgan, Michael, *Optimum Sports Nutrition*, Advance Research Press, New York,1993

Consensus Development Conference on Insulin Resistance. November 5-6, 1997. American Diabetes Association. Diabetes Care 1998;21:310-4.

deLemos, M.L., *Effects of soy phytoestrogens genistein and daidzein on breast cancer growth*, Am Pharmacother, 35:1118- 1121, 2001

Divi, R.L., et al, *Anti-thyroid isoflavones from soybeans: isolation, characterization, and mechanisms of action*, Biochem Pharmacol, 54:1087-1096,1997

Fairfield MD Dr Ph, K. and Fletcher MD MSc, R.H. *"Vitamins for Chronic Disease Prevention in Adults"*. JAMA 2002; 287: Pp. 3116-3126, 3127-3129.

Food Label.(www.cfsan.fda.gov/~dms/foodlab.html). How to Understand and Use the Nutrition Facts Label. US FDA, 2004.

Glycemic Index. (www.glycemicindex.com).

Harris, MI, et al (1998) *Prevalence of diabetes, impaired fasting glucose, and impaired glucose tolerance in US adults*. The Third National Health and Nutrition Examination Survey, 19988-1994 Diabetes Care, 21, 518-524

Havel PJ. *Update on adipocyte hormones: regulation of energy balance and carbohydrate/lipid metabolism*. Diabetes 2004;53(Suppl. 1):S143-51.

HESSLINK, R Jr, et al. Cetylated Fatty Acids Improve Knee Function in Patients with Osteoarthritis. J Rheumatol 2002;29:1708-12.

Jazet IM, Pijl H, Meinders AE. *Adipose tissue as an endocrine organ: impact on insulin resistance*. Neth J Med 2003;61(6):194-212.

Jellin JM, Batz F, Hitchens K. Pharmacist's Letter/Prescriber's Letter Natural Medicines Comprehensive Database. Stockton, CA: Therapeutic Research Faculty; 2003 (available as textbook, CD and online)

Murkies, A. et al, *Phytoestrogens and breast cancer in postmenopausal women: a case control study*, Menopause, 7:289-296, 2000

Jenkins DJ, Kendall CW, Axelsen M, Augustin LS, Vuksan V. *Viscous and nonviscous fibres, nonabsorbable and low glycaemic index carbohydrates, blood lipids and coronary heart disease*. Curr Opin Lipidol 2000;11:49-56.

LaValle, J.B. *Natural Therapeutics Pocket Guide*. 2000. Lexi-Comp. Hudson, OH. Pg. 680.

Laville M, Cornu C, Normand S, et al. *Decreased glucose-induced thermogenesis at the onset of obesity*. Am J Clin Nutr 1993;57:851-856.

Lin B.H., C.L. Huang and S.A. French (2004). *"Factors associated with women's and children's body mass indices by income status,"* International J. Obesity 28:536-43.

Lissin, L.W., Cooke, J.P., *Phytoestrogens and cardiovascular health*, J Am Coll Cardiol, 35:1403-1410, 2000

Massey, L.K., et al, *Oxalate content of soybean seeds (Glycine max. Leguminosae), soyfoods, and other edible legumes*, J Agric Foods, 49:4262-4266, 2001

Matthews, Dwight E., *Proteins and Amino Acids*, in Maurice E Shils, James A. Olson, Moshe Shike, A Catharine Ross, editors, Modern Nutrition In Health and Disease, ninth edition, Lippincott Williams & Wilkins New York,1999

Mendosa, D. (www.mendosa.com/common_foods_bw.htm). Glycemic Values of Common American Foods. 2003.

Middlemost, M. www.phoenixfitness.ca.

Murphy, J. Michael EdD; Wehler, Cheryl A. MS; Pagano, Maria E. EdM; Little, Michelle BA; Kleinman, Ronald E. MD; Jellinek, Micheal S. MD. *"Relationship Between Hunger and Psychosocial Functioning in Low-Income American Children"*, Journal of the American Academy of Child and Adolescent Psychiatry, February, 1998.

Murray, M., www.doctormurray.com.

Ogden CL, Fryar CD, Carroll MD, Flegal KM. *Mean bodyweight, height, and body mass index,* United States 1960–2002. Advance data from vital and health statistics; no347. Hyattsville, Maryland: National Center for Health Statistics.2004.

Pizzorno, J., Murray, M. Textbook of Natural Medicine. London, UK: Churchill Livingstone, 2000.

Potter, S.M., et al, *Soy protein and isoflavones: their effects on blood lipids and bone density in postmenopausal women,* Am J clin Nutr, 68(Suppl):1375s-1379s,1998

Prochaska, J., Norcross, J., DiCLemente, C. *Changing for Good.* New York, NY: Avon Books Inc, 1994.

Ravussin E, Acheson KJ, Vernet O et al. *Evidence that insulin resistance is responsible for the decreased thermic effect of glucose in human obesity.* J Clin Invest 1985; 76: 1268-1273

Schils ME., et al. Modern Nutrition in Health and Disease. Baltimore, MD: Lippincott Wiliams & Wilkins. 1999.

Setchell, Kenneth, et al, *Dietary Isoflavones: Biological effects and relevance to human health,* J Nutr, 129 (Suppl):758s- 767s, 1999

Statistics Canada – *The Daily.* Tuesday, June 15, 2004. Canadian Community Health Survey

Steinberger J, Moran A, Hong CP, Jacobs DR Jr, Sinaiko AR. *"Adiposity in childhood predicts obesity and insulin resistance in young adulthood",* Journal of Pediatrics April 2001.

US Census Bureau, *Population Estimates,* 2004

US Census Bureau, *International Data Base,* 2004

Vuksan V, Lyon M, Breitman P, Sievenpiper J. *3-Week Consumption of a Highly Viscous Dietary Fibre Blend Results in Improvements in Insulin Sensitivity and Reductions in Body Fat. Results of a double blind, placebo controlled trial.* Presented at the 64th Annual Meeting of the American Diabetes Association. Orlando, Florida; June 4-8, 2004.

Diabetes Care 2000;23:9-14.

Warren,Janet M. PhD; Henry, C. Jeya K. PhD; Simonite Vanessa, PhD. *"Low Glycemic Index Breakfasts and Reduced Food Intake in Preadolescent Children"*, PEDIATRICS November 2003.

Wright, J.V. and Gaby, A. *The Patient's Book of Natural Healing.* 1999. Prima Health. Rocklin, CA. Pp. xii, 388.

Vuksan V, Jenkins DJ, Spadafora P, et al. *Konjac-mannan (glucomannan) improves glycemia and other associated risk factors for coronary heart disease in type 2 diabetes. A randomized controlled metabolic trial.* Diabetes Care 1999;22:913-9.

Vuksan V, Sievenpiper JL, Owen R, et al. *Beneficial effects of viscous dietary fiber from Konjac-mannan in subjects with the insulin resistance syndrome: results of a controlled metabolic trial.* Diabetes Care 2000;23:9-14.

Illustration Credits

pp 3, 42, 69, 80, 85 .... Gerry Apuada

p 5.. John Jonik

p 7.. Nick Kim

p 52 .... John Trever

Daily Journal

Carry a notebook, or use a chart like this to record everything you eat and drink.

MONDAY

Breakfast

Snack

Lunch

Snack

Dinner

Snack

TUESDAY

Breakfast

Snack

Lunch

Snack

Dinner

Snack

WEDNESDAY

Breakfast

Snack

Lunch

Snack

Dinner

Snack

THURSDAY

Breakfast

Snack

Lunch

Snack

Dinner

Snack

FRIDAY

Breakfast

Snack

Lunch

Snack

Dinner

Snack

SATURDAY

Breakfast

Snack

Lunch

Snack

Dinner

Snack

SUNDAY

Breakfast

Snack

Lunch

Snack

Dinner

Snack

Goal Chart

Chart your progress. In the exercise and nutrition columns, write your goals for the week. Be as specific as possible. At the end of the week evaluate yourself with a (**+**) if you achieved or surpassed your goal, and a (**–**) if you did not.

	Exercise Goal	+/-	Nutrition Goal	+/-
Week 1				
Week 2				
Week 3				
Week 4				
Week 5				
Week 6				
Week 7				
Week 8				
Week 9				
Week 10				
Week 11				
Week 12				

	Exercise Goal	+/-	Nutrition Goal	+/-
Week 13				
Week 14				
Week 15				
Week 16				
Week 17				
Week 18				
Week 19				
Week 20				
Week 21				
Week 22				
Week 23				
Week 24